T0239281

# So You Want to Teach Clinical?

Teaching nursing students in a clinical setting with patients differs greatly from teaching in a classroom. It can be a daunting task if one is not prepared and mentored.

This book provides a concise and accessible guide for nursing instructors leading students in the healthcare agency for the first time, as well as experienced educators who are interested in exploring new teaching strategies. It covers many aspects of the clinical instructor role including:

- meeting the nurse manager
- organizing and documenting your clinical day
- creating clinical student assignments
- objectively evaluating student's individual performance
- acknowledging diversity and inclusiveness
- tracking progress and handling student errors

In addition, the book discusses some of the more complex issues surrounding the role of the clinical instructor such as accountability for nursing care, documentation and medication administration carried out by students.

The book features numerous forms and charts to assist in organizing and managing the teaching experience, as well as situational scenarios to help prepare instructors for unique situations that arise during the clinical experience.

Written by authors with extensive experience in clinical care and teaching, this book will be an invaluable guide for all clinical nursing instructors, both novice and experienced.

**Laura A. Jaroneski** is currently an adjunct nursing faculty member at Macomb Community College. Her clinical experience spans 25 years as a medical-surgical and oncology staff nurse plus 14 years as nursing faculty teaching students to critically think in didactic courses, clinical settings, skills assessment laboratories and high-fidelity patient simulations.

**Lori A. Przymusinski**, a nurse for 35 years, focused her career on the care of adult medical surgical patients. She became a full-time nursing faculty member at Oakland Community College in 2006, lecturing and leading students through their clinical experiences for 12 years, where she later served as the Dean and Associate Dean of Nursing and Health Professions for four years, guiding the program's eight-year reaccreditation from the Accreditation Commission for Education in Nursing (ACEN) in 2014.

LAURA A. JARONESKI AND
LORI A. PRZYMUSINSKI

# So You Want to Teach Clinical?

## A Guide for New Nursing Clinical Instructors

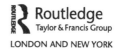

Routledge
Taylor & Francis Group

LONDON AND NEW YORK

First published 2019
by Routledge
2 Park Square, Milton Park, Abingdon, Oxon OX14 4RN

and by Routledge
711 Third Avenue, New York, NY 10017

*Routledge is an imprint of the Taylor & Francis Group, an informa business*

*British Library Cataloguing-in-Publication Data*
A catalogue record for this book is available from the British Library

*Library of Congress Cataloging-in-Publication Data*

Names: Jaroneski, Laura A., author. | Przymusinski, Lori A., author.
Title: So you want to teach clinical? : a guide for new clinical instructors /
    Laura A. Jaroneski and Lori A. Przymusinski.
Description: Abingdon, Oxon ; New York, NY : Routledge, 2019. |
    Includes bibliographical references and index.
Identifiers: LCCN 2018025639| ISBN 9781138616257 (hardback) |
    ISBN 9781138616264 (pbk.) | ISBN 9780429462320 (ebook)
Subjects: | MESH: Education, Nursing—methods | Teaching | Clinical Competence
Classification: LCC RT73 | NLM WY 18 | DDC 610.73071/1—dc23
LC record available at https://lccn.loc.gov/2018025639

ISBN: 978-1-138-61625-7 (hbk)
ISBN: 978-1-138-61626-4 (pbk)
ISBN: 978-0-429-46232-0 (ebk)

Typeset in Joanna MT and Din
by Apex CoVantage, LLC

Visit the eResource: www.routledge.com/9781138616264

This book is dedicated to our spouses Jack Jaroneski and Dean Przymusinski for their patience during our writing journey.

# Contents

This book was written to assist new nursing instructors. We know that sometimes nurses decide to take on this role and discover it involves a great deal of preparation and time. This guide is structured to help you plan your first, and subsequent, clinical teaching assignments. Our hope is that even seasoned clinical instructors will benefit from the information provided. Numerous examples with instructions for use will be presented throughout the book to assist you with organizing the clinical rotation and documenting its progression. These forms will allow you to fairly assess each student's performance and provide a final evaluation. The book is set up in sequential order starting with the information about the clinical nursing role and program information, preparing for clinical, managing the actual clinical day concluding with student evaluation guidance. Along the way pertinent information, which we hope you will find valuable, including critical thinking, alternative experiences, diversity, collaboration and collegiality, is discussed.

The first chapter welcomes you to the realm of clinical teaching. While teaching students is a very different experience than providing bedside nursing care, a comparison is made between the two roles. It is quite possible you are hired very near the beginning of a semester with minimal time to prepare for this exciting opportunity. The chapter begins to lay a foundation for you, starting with basic information about the nursing program curriculum. Nursing program and course learning goals are developed so you can have a road map during the clinical rotation. As a gatekeeper for the nursing profession you must observe safe behaviors and evidence of learned knowledge from all students to determine if they have met the minimum requirements to continue to the next level, or graduation. Influential entities drive the quality of nursing programs and accreditation standards must also be included in the teaching curriculum. There are several organizations like the American Nurses Association (ANA), Quality and Safety Education in Nursing (QSEN) and accrediting agencies that guide nursing programs to design their curricula. You will be continuously prioritizing, assessing, delegating and guiding students to assure the patients you assign to them remain safe during your watch. Clinical teaching is far from easy but is a very rewarding and important job!

Chapter Two provides information for you to make a smooth transition into the realm of clinical teaching. You will learn about the role of the lead faculty and how they are very a valuable resource for additional information and support. We also provide information about the initial clinical agency visit prior to your clinical start. Meeting the nurse manager, familiarizing yourself with the agency policies and procedures and completion of any mandatory competencies is an important step in preparation for your first clinical day.

You will soon realize as you assume the instructor role you will be more scrutinized as a role model for the nursing profession. Chapter Three discusses how your demonstration of professionalism and ethical standards will set the tone for your instructor-student relationship. Professional expectations of the students are discussed along with tips on promoting proper communication and use of technology in the clinical setting.

Chapter Four presents a thorough explanation of how to organize student orientation to the agency and manage subsequent clinical days. Reflection of clinical situations and work flow encountered during a clinical experience should be anticipated prior to the start of the experience. Advice about how to determine student assignments, facilitate communication during the shift, reviewing the goals for student learning using course objectives, and documentation in the electronic medical record is provided. Information on post-conference is also presented. Your primary role as an instructor is to monitor student progress, despite the distractions you will encounter on a busy nursing unit. Tools to record your observations are included in this chapter to provide you with templates to document fair and accurate assessment of students' performance. We know you will find them helpful.

The clinical guide would not be complete without a discussion about critical thinking, which is highlighted in Chapter Five. Much has been published, discussed, and examined about critical thinking and its importance for nursing education. New educators may wish to spend time reviewing these resources to familiarize themselves with ways to measure student "thinking" in a nursing care encounter. In this chapter we provide several examples outlining ways to evaluate a student's critical thinking. Concept maps, which provide a way for students to display their critical thinking about an assigned patient illustrating their diagnosis, nursing interventions, health care team interactions and rationale for the care provided are a great learning tool! A sample of a completed concept map is included among the provided examples for a better understanding of this assignment.

Medication administration by students and supervised by you, as discussed in Chapter Six, is extensively covered. Although you may be uneasy about letting students give medications to patients, and it is a complex challenge, we have presented the process in segments, so you will feel more confident as you oversee them. Utilizing pertinent questioning skills to assess a student's knowledge will help you to determine a student's readiness to administer medications. Following our suggestions will increase your confidence in this task, and fully alert you to students who may not be prepared to give medications, ultimately allowing you to protect a patient from an unfortunate error! We also have included several forms to assist you with documenting student progress in this specific realm.

In Chapter Seven alternative experiences for nursing students that may be utilized to enhance learning during a clinical day are presented. It is mandatory, however, that you check with the lead nursing faculty before sending students to any of them! Alternative assignments and experiences that relate to clinical course objectives might be included in your overall performance evaluation of the student at the end of the semester. If approved, some ideas for alternative experiences and assignments are presented for consideration. A written summary of the experience to be submitted to you by the participating student is recommended to add value to an alternative assignment. Each instructor should be able to identify alternative experience opportunities depending on the agency but must always follow the guidance provided by the program. You want to ensure that the student's time is productive and well spent!

Acknowledgement of diversity and inclusiveness is a vital skill in health care. Chapter Eight guides you through some unfamiliar situations that students will encounter. The patient population at the agency where you are teaching clinical usually reflects the cultural and ethnic composition of the surrounding community. Informing students about practices that may occur among specific groups in advance will help them feel more confident. Specific topics and examples that are discussed in this chapter include student and staff diversity, gender and sexual orientation, religious practices, and customs surrounding death and dying.

The concise and fair evaluation of students is one of the most important tasks you must accomplish as a clinical instructor, as discussed in Chapter Nine. You must determine if each student has demonstrated knowledge of safe practice to proceed along, or graduate from the nursing program. We know it is a big responsibility but anticipating a student failure should begin prior to you meeting a clinical group for the first time. You may hope that a struggling student improves with more practice in their next clinical rotation and want to pass them along, but your job is to provide them with resources for improvement. Skills remediation processes are presented so that students can have the best chance for success. They rely on concise documentation, and communication with the nursing program lead faculty. Throughout the book, the examples we have provided, if used by you, will allow you to evaluate each student and summarize your observations collectively. A final evaluation tool is included if you need it. Additional guidance will be offered about how to prepare documentation, acquire support, and deliver news of a failure to a student, which can be a very uncomfortable encounter!

Just as in your role as a staff nurse, a clinical nursing instructor must collaborate with the staff at the agency. You will face some questions and concerns as you begin this new experience! In Chapter Ten we provide answers to help you feel more at ease with the new situations you may encounter in this role. It is important to remember that you are not alone and there are many resources and professionals available to guide you on this journey. You also have an essential accountability to the agency and patient safety. Incivility, bullying and lateral violence, which we hope you will not encounter, are presented, so that you may be prepared to manage them if you do! Your focus on nursing practice which is collaborative and collegial will build positive rapport and trust and will benefit yourself and your students now and in the future.

Carry our guide to clinical with you. We have tried to think of everything that we wish we had known when we first started out! The forms that we have referenced in the text are downloadable from the publisher's website and will truly help you to succeed, and refine your organizational skills, as you move on to future clinical assignments. We hope that our 25 plus years of clinical teaching experience will provide you with extensive support as you venture into this new realm of nursing. Preparing the next generation of nurses is important and rewarding. Witnessing former students that you have mentored, working as practicing nurses, is awesome. We hope you discover the same passion for teaching clinical nursing that we have. Welcome!

Best regards,
Laura and Lori

# Acknowledgement

We wish to acknowledge the creativity of Judith Przymusinski, our graphic artist, who designed the forms that we believe are the heart of the book. They will truly guide a new or experienced clinical instructor to organize and conduct a successful teaching experience.

# Abbreviations

| | |
|---|---|
| ACEN | Accreditation Commission for Education in Nursing |
| ANA | American Nurses Association |
| BP | Blood pressure |
| BS | Blood sugar |
| BSO | Bilateral Salingo-Oophorectomy |
| CBC | Complete blood count |
| CCNE | Commission on Collegiate Nursing Education |
| CMS | Centers for Medicare and Medicaid Services |
| CPP | Clinical Proficiency and Progression tool |
| CT | Computed tomography |
| EMR | Electronic medical record |
| ETOH | Ethyl alcohol, used to describe an individual's abuse |
| FBS | Fasting blood sugar |
| FERPA | Family Educational Rights and Privacy Act |
| HIPAA | Health Insurance Portability and Accountability Act |
| IV | Intravenous |
| LGBTQ | Lesbian, Gay, Bisexual, Transgender, Queer |
| MAR | Medication Administration Record |
| NA | Nursing assistant |
| NGT | Nasogastric tube |
| NLN | National League for Nursing |
| OR | Operating room |
| PACU | Post anesthesia care unit |

| | |
|---|---|
| PaO$_2$ | Arterial partial pressure of oxygen |
| PCT | Patient care technician |
| PRN | As needed |
| QSEN | Quality and Safety Education for Nurses |
| TAH | Total Abdominal Hysterectomy |
| TIA | Transient ischemic attack |
| TJC | The Joint Commission |
| TPN | Total parenteral nutrition |
| TURP | Transurethral resection of the prostate |
| UAP | Unlicensed assistive personnel |

# Author biographies

**Laura A. Jaroneski** earned her BSN and MSN Ed degrees from Oakland University in Rochester, Michigan. Most of her nursing career was spent working at a mid-sized community hospital with adult medical-surgical patients. She eventually specialized as an oncology nurse and obtained oncology nurse certification (OCN). After obtaining her MSN she worked as full-time nursing faculty at Baker College in Clinton Township, Michigan, and currently is an adjunct faculty member at Macomb Community College in Clinton Township, Michigan.

As nursing faculty, Laura Jaroneski has taught across the curriculum in a variety of settings to include medical-surgical didactic courses, clinical nursing, fundamental and health assessment skills labs, and high-fidelity patient simulations. As lead faculty for her courses she was also involved in curriculum revisions, counseling of nursing students on learning strategies, and critical thinking and mentoring new clinical nursing faculty.

Laura Jaroneski's professional recognitions include:

- 2003 – The Oncology Nurse Recognition Award
- 2012 – Daisy Faculty Award

She has been published in *Oncology Times*, *Oncology Nursing*

Forum, the *Metropolitan Detroit Oncology Nursing Society Chapter Capsule* and *Teaching and Learning in Nursing*. She has written and revised the instructor's PowerPoint presentations for a gerontological nursing textbook and written ten chapters in a pharmacology nursing textbook on student learning strategies.

Professional memberships include the National League of Nursing (NLN) and the Oncology Nursing Society (ONS).

**Lori A. Przymusinski** earned a certificate of Practical Nursing and Associate Degree in Applied Science at Oakland Community College, Waterford, Michigan. She completed her BSN at Oakland University in Rochester, Michigan, and her MSN at the University of Phoenix, Detroit campus. She worked as a staff nurse, manager, clinical nurse specialist and administrative nursing supervisor for a large teaching hospital system in southeastern Michigan. Her acute care experience focused on general surgical patients including the areas of neurology, orthopedics, urology and renal-hemodialysis.

After a 20-year acute care career Lori Przymusinski pursued teaching nursing in higher education. She served as an adjunct instructor, and later full-time faculty member, in the Associate Degree nursing program at Baker College Clinton Township, Michigan, and Oakland Community College, Waterford, and Southfield, Michigan. Her clinical and theory teaching included the areas of Fundamentals of Nursing, Advanced Medical-Surgical: Orthopedics and Neurology, Pharmacology and Nursing Leadership. At Oakland Community College she had extensive experience in course and curriculum development. In 2011 she became the Dean of Nursing and Health Professions at Oakland Community College, and in 2014 facilitated the eight-year reaccreditation of the Associate Degree nursing program by the Accreditation Commission for Education in Nursing (ACEN). Since 2017 Lori has been the Vice Chancellor for Student Services at Oakland Community College.

Lori Przymusinski's professional recognitions include:

- 1998 – Oakland University Board of Visitors Award-recognition of an outstanding RN-BSN completion student
- 2011 – Outstanding Faculty of the Year, Oakland Community College
- 2014 – University of Phoenix, Detroit campus Alumni of the Year

She has been published in *The Humanist* and the former *RN Excellence* Michigan, a statewide publication for nurses. She has also been a reviewer for several pharmacology publications.

Professional memberships include a sustaining membership in the National Student Nurses' Association (NSNA), and the Michigan Nurses Association (MNA).

# One

Congratulations! As the result of your credentials and knowledge, you have been selected to teach nursing students. Clinical teaching is far from easy, but is a very rewarding and important job. To assist you with organizing the clinical rotation and documenting its progression, we provide numerous forms throughout the book that you can download. Several completed examples are in the Appendices.

Although you successfully completed a nursing program, teaching students is a very different experience than providing bedside nursing care. As a first-time clinical instructor, it is possible you are hired near the beginning of a semester with minimal time to learn or to prepare for this exciting opportunity. Now, not only are you thinking about patient care and good outcomes, but you will also guide inexperienced individuals to the same type of thinking! It is very gratifying to witness a nursing student's "aha" moment that you know you created with your expert knowledge and support. It is an even greater delight to see them graduate and later encounter them in practice as a peer!

Teaching, although a major expectation of your role, is not the only activity you will be focusing on. You will be continuously prioritizing, assessing, delegating and guiding students to assure the patients you assign to them remain safe during your clinical day. Nurses teach patients and significant others about disease management and care to support positive results. Nursing instructors provide the same teaching to students at a more complex level but with the same intended goal.

### NURSING PROGRAM OVERVIEW

Each nursing program must have learning outcomes that describe the expected student behaviors in each clinical experience. The program curriculum is constructed using tenets developed by a nursing theorist(s) that guide the learning objectives and are embraced by the program—both in the classroom and clinical. This is true for any level of nursing program: Practical nurse, associate degree, and baccalaureate. The course syllabus serves as a contract between you and the student in the event they fail to meet clinical course outcomes, as discussed in later chapters. The contents of this book can be adapted for any program and any level of student that you are leading.

Nursing program curriculum moves in an upward direction, course by course, requiring more complex knowledge and skill acquisition by the student as they move through a program. Students must draw on previous learned information and apply it to new experiences in the classroom, laboratory, and clinical setting. From the initial nursing fundamental course to the senior capstone experience, learning outcomes will align with behaviors and skills that the student must demonstrate by course conclusion.

Patricia Benner (1984) describes this progression from novice to expert in nursing education that encompasses an individual's transition into the role of a practicing professional nurse. Her theory concludes that this growth will continue several years post-graduation with oversight assumed by experienced nurses and nursing managers who will guide a novice nurse's integration as a professional nurse.

Nursing program and course learning goals are designed to be measurable. The outcomes developed for clinical evaluation of a student are predominantly qualitative. As a clinical instructor and gatekeeper for the profession, you must observe these behaviors by all students during your clinical interaction to determine if they have met the minimum requirements to continue to the next level, or graduation. Recognizing this, it becomes your responsibility to familiarize yourself with the course syllabus, so you can accurately evaluate all student performance. It can feel overwhelming and it is not unusual to doubt yourself as you evolve into this new role.

## ACCREDITATION AND PROFESSIONAL NURSING ORGANIZATIONS

In a health care agency, The Joint Commission (TJC) and the Centers for Medicare and Medicaid Services (CMS) are organizations that provide acknowledgement of quality for an agency. These accreditation standards guide a health care agency towards the development of quality operations to achieve measurable, excellent patient care outcomes. In a similar way, standards and accreditation drive the quality of nursing programs which must be included in the curriculum. The American Nurses Association (ANA) is the professional organization from which nursing programs derive standards that all nurses in practice must exhibit. These may be viewed on the ANA website http://www.nursingworld.org.

Accrediting agencies specifically focused on nursing education quality expect students are educated and prepared to begin nursing practice with the most current knowledge base. Accredited nursing programs are reviewed on a cyclic schedule-every five to eight years. Not all programs have accreditation.

Accrediting agencies include: Commission on Collegiate Nursing Education (CCNE), the Accreditation Commission for Education in Nursing (ACEN), and the National League for Nursing (NLN). Information about the specific expectations for program accreditation may be found on their websites. If the accreditation cycle occurs while you are teaching, you could be asked to participate in a review, particularly when you become experienced and successful in your clinical teaching endeavors!

The Quality and Safety Education for Nurses (QSEN) Institute is a collaborative of healthcare professionals dedicated to improving the quality and safety of health care systems. Nursing schools are including the QSEN competencies in their curriculum to prepare future nurses to recognize deficiencies and improve the quality and safety of the healthcare system. QSEN defines pre-licensure and graduate quality and safety competencies for nursing students (QSEN.org, 2018). Courses in a nursing program increase in difficulty and build on previously learned knowledge. Assignments that demonstrate proficiency at the student's level of knowledge may be used by you to measure their grasp of the information. Chapter Seven details clinical activities that support QSEN to include in your clinical teaching.

### REFERENCES

Accreditation Commission for Education in Nursing (ACEN). http://www.acenursing.org/

American Nurses Association (ANA). http://www.nursingworld.org

Benner, P. (1984). *From novice to expert, excellence and power in clinical nursing practice.* Addison Wesley, Menlo Park, CA.

Centers for Medicare and Medicaid Services (CMS). http://www.cms.gov.

Commission on Collegiate Nursing Education (CCNE). http://www.aacnnursing.org/CCNE

National League for Nursing (NLN). http://www.nln.org/

Quality and Safety Education for Nurses (QSEN). http://qsen.org

The Joint Commission (TJC). https://jointcommission.org

# **Two**

Nurses are trained to be methodical thinkers. The escalation of a nurse's responsibility in a continually complex healthcare environment requires pre-planning and organization on a shift-by-shift basis. In your professional practice, during a hand-off report you analyze the priority assessments, interventions and begin planning to assure your assigned patients will receive safe and quality care.

As an experienced professional nurse, you are accustomed to managing your own practice independently. Oversight for a group of inexperienced novices in a clinical rotation is very different. You are responsible not only for the patients you may assign to the students, but for the students *and* their actions. Clinical teaching multiplies your professional accountability to these patients and the health care agency. Planning your strategy for this challenge as a clinical instructor ahead of time allows you to focus on the fast-paced clinical days you will experience. We have provided a checklist to guide you in obtaining important details related to your clinical assignment. Receipt of the syllabus, contact information of lead faculty and agency orientation dates and times are examples of activities that must be completed prior to the start of your first clinical rotation. Form 2A Pre-Semester Preparation/ Checklist for Clinical Teaching can assist you. We suggest compiling a binder at the start of each clinical assignment, so all relevant information can be readily available to you for reference.

## NURSING PROGRAM LEADERSHIP

We cannot stress enough the importance of establishing an open line of communication with the lead faculty or coordinator of the nursing program where you teach. Lead faculty oversee the curriculum both in and out of the classroom and will familiarize you with the educational outcomes of the program. They are content experts and have substantial input into the syllabus. They are also your lifeline if you encounter barriers to achieving the outcomes for students during the clinical rotation. Changes in expectations or student policies imposed by the clinical agency, handling student conduct such as policy breaches, or guidance when you identify that a student may not successfully complete your clinical rotation are examples. Clinical failure is discussed in Chapter Nine.

Attendance at a nursing program orientation and clinical course meetings, if offered, are strongly encouraged. There may be a pre, midterm and post-semester meeting you may be expected to attend. Interacting with the lead faculty and other instructors is evidence of your commitment to your new role as a clinical educator. Networking with these individuals will also provide you with ideas about how to address difficulties you may encounter during a clinical day and will open lines of communication. You may be working in another nursing position, but academic calendars are established early in the year permitting you to plan for your attendance.

## VISITING THE CLINICAL SITE

Many clinical agencies require a mandatory orientation annually for all clinical instructors. It is also highly recommended, and may be required, to meet with the nurse manager of the nursing unit where you will bring your clinical group. Initiating this relationship will allow you to become familiar to the manager, while providing you with an opportunity to share the student's skill level and course outcomes. The manager may provide unit information and direct you to resources you will need to be successful, such as hospital policies and procedures. A nurse educator or clinical nurse specialist can be an invaluable resource as well, and can alert you to educational opportunities for your group to experience. We recommend spending a minimum of one half-day on the nursing unit shadowing a staff nurse to obtain a firsthand experience of a typical day. This relationship building provides an excellent opportunity for communication of expectations from both the clinical agency and academic viewpoints, which will enhance your reputation as a professional. As experienced clinical instructors, we became very recognizable to the managers and staff we encountered. Over time we were considered part of the team, as were the students we taught, and so will you.

### STUDENT PLACEMENT IN CLINICAL SITES

Student clinical placements at agency sites are assigned in different ways. Placement can vary by state and sometimes by the nursing agencies. Some states utilize a centralized clinical placement program to create equal opportunity for nursing programs to secure placing their students in preferred clinical sites. Many times, clinical sites are utilized by clinical groups from other nursing schools and universities throughout the week. Therefore, it is very important to arrange the manager meeting a few weeks in advance.

Every clinical agency has their own set of required mandatory competencies and preparations for all instructors and students to complete prior to the first day of clinical. These may include any or all of the following: blood-borne pathogen training, fire safety, infection control, confidentiality and computer access training. In many states there are centralized clinical consortiums that may provide computer training modules on these topics. This training may be annual, but agency specific competencies may also be required. If agency specific competencies are required, schedule them on the first day so it becomes part of orientation day. Information on orientation day is discussed in Chapter Four. Students will also need training on the use of the electronic medical record (EMR) documentation system. It is up to the instructor to arrange for the training or train the students themselves.

---

**AUTHORS' TIP**

Purchase a small notebook that will fit in your pocket to carry with you on the unit. Use it to keep all the important phone numbers handy for the clinical. Examples include the unit desk, the nurse manager, the pharmacy, and the contact personnel for any of the following: security, nursing education, clinical nurse specialist or contact person at your college.

Role modeling and professional expectations

# Three

As mentioned earlier, you are an expert nurse. You are also aware that nursing continues to be one of the most respected professions many years running, as reported by several large polling groups. With this responsibility comes the expectation that you will present yourself professionally and possess high ethical standards. Remember you may be teaching at a new agency where no one knows you and you only have one chance to make a great first impression. Managers and staff notice your demeanor and how you interact with your clinical group. They will conclude that you, and your students, are representative of the nursing program you are working for and will note this as they approve future clinical site requests. Despite all your efforts, you cannot choose the students you will be assigned to lead into the clinical experience. Here are a few suggestions for your consideration to assist with setting parameters and addressing student needs to support a successful experience.

## RELATIONSHIP BUILDING WITH STUDENTS

Professionalism and ethics are qualities that you must role model to your nursing students during your interactions with them privately and in front of their peers, patients, and other agency personnel. Nursing programs admit a variety of individuals to programs who come from many backgrounds and age groups. Depending on their values and previous experiences they will initially view you as their "supervisor" of the clinical experience, and a guide to their continued success. It is your responsibility to maintain that professional relationship even though you will have students who may be older than you or possess different or unfamiliar value systems from yours.

During your first meeting on orientation day, state to the students how you wish to be addressed ie: Mrs., Mr., Dr., or by your first name. Students who are older than you may be respectful of your position, or may view you as inexperienced, even though they are novices about nursing practice themselves. They may view and address you from a matriarchal or patriarchal level if you are a similar age of their own child or other family member. Likewise, students who are nearer to your age may attempt to develop some familiarity with you as a peer even though you are in a role of authority. Your goal is to develop an instructor-student relationship, remain professional, and treat all students equally.

### STUDENT DEMOGRAPHICS

It is highly likely that you will lead a clinical group consisting of students who are from different generations and possess varying skills and social values. More information about diversity is discussed in Chapter Eight. However, when trying to evaluate the need of your group some considerations must be acknowledged. Chronological age will impact a student's knowledge of technology, their stamina, manual dexterity, and possible academic success. Life experiences students bring to the clinical setting may also be influential. Nursing may be a second career choice for individuals who have experienced job dissatisfaction or loss due to economics.

Teaching a diverse group of students can be challenging but is far from impossible if you gather information about them on the first day.

Using your assessment skills, you can identify and prioritize immediate needs for some members of the group as you begin the clinical experience. You may not get to know all of your students at once. Students may share personal and academic information with you as your clinical progresses.

### COMMUNICATION WHILE ON THE NURSING UNIT

Continue to remind students that they are in a professional setting where order, civility, and confidentiality are necessary to assure excellent nursing care is being provided. Students must learn who their resources are and develop and practice familiarity with acceptable methods of communicating. Establish ground rules for communication methods on the first day with the group so they may contact you if they require assistance. Assure that they identify each day who the agency staff is that they can reach out to if you are not immediately available to respond to them. Raising voices, yelling down a hall, and making sudden wild gestures is not professional behavior. This can be misinterpreted as a true emergency by other staff members.

The use of technology and personal devices must also have specific parameters. Texting, taking photographs and making personal phone calls in the patient care area must be prohibited. Use of the EMR is limited to researching and documenting information related to students' assigned patients only. Privacy protocol dictates compliance to the Health Insurance Portability and Accountability Act (HIPAA).

Remind students that communication with patients and their significant others must remain professional and must surround the plan of care. It must always be pleasant, articulate, and brief. Lengthy discussions about personal medical or hospital experiences, complaints about the agency, personnel, or nursing school experiences must not occur. You will be notified if you have a student engaging in this type of interaction. Examples of non-therapeutic communication behaviors should be documented in your notes during the evaluation of the student.

Setting high expectations for professionalism early during clinical with every interaction will create habits that students can carry into their future careers with your guidance.

### SCENARIO 3-1 NON-THERAPEUTIC COMMUNICATION ENCOUNTER

You are leading a clinical group on a Women's Health unit and have assigned Cindy to care for a 38-year-old female patient on the first post-operative day after a Total Abdominal Hysterectomy (TAH) and Bilateral Salpingo-Oophorectomy (BSO) due to a history of cystic fibroid disease. Cindy is very close to the age of the patient. You overhear from the doorway the student stating to the patient "Do you already have children?" The patient bursts into tears. Your actions in this situation will include:

- Immediately enter the room, introduce yourself to the patient, and offer any comfort measures.
- Assess the patient's pain level.
- Assess if her emotional reaction is due to the student's statement.
- If pain intervention is requested, arrange for it to be provided by the assigned nurse.
- Remove the student from the room.
- Inform the nurse of the interaction.

- Meet privately with the student to review the verbal exchange. Assess:

  o The student's efforts to research the assigned patient's diagnosis.
  o The student's awareness of their non-therapeutic statement and awareness about the use of empathy.

- Reassign the student to a new patient.
- Document the encounter anecdotally for your notes; provide a written summary to the student of their deficient performance using the evaluation tool in the syllabus or the *Clinical Proficiency and Progression* (CPP) tool in Form 9A as a guide. The student in this encounter does not meet criteria for "Exhibits therapeutic nurse-patient relationship building skills…"
- Consult with the lead faculty to determine a plan for remediation.
- Continue to document your observations of the student and note if improvement occurs during student nurse-patient interactions.

### SCENARIO 3-2 BREACH OF PROTECTED PATIENT INFORMATION

At the end of the clinical day you observe a student in your clinical group, Julie, at the nurses' station printing many pages. Upon review you note that this is protected information including the history and physical notes, laboratory values, and the results of radiologic studies from the EMR about her assigned patient. The student notes that you are approaching and states "I am getting updated information about my patient, so I can compare to yesterday's lab results".

Further investigation reveals that Julie printed similar information the previous day and took it home to review and begin completing a nursing care plan assignment. You will:

- Instruct Julie to cease printing any more documents and direct her to discard the ones she previously printed (if she has them) in the shredding receptacle.
- Speak to the student privately and review the privacy guidelines that were reviewed on the first day of clinical.
- Assess if the student understands the professional and legal expectation of health care professionals to abide by HIPAA that is federally mandated.
- Document anecdotally the encounter. Provide the student with a copy of a written summary of the discussion and agency expectations for handling private patient information.
- Refer the student to the Clinical Proficiency and Progression (CPP) tool Form 9A, or the evaluation tool used in their course syllabi, to advise them that this incident does not meet the course objectives.
- Notify the lead faculty of the incident for further guidance and action.

Organizing and documenting your clinical day

# Four

### CLINICAL ORIENTATION DAY

The first day of clinical is the time to provide the students with your expectations and how you plan for the clinical days to be structured. If an instructor appears organized, the students will generally follow their lead. Providing an orientation that includes a tour of the nursing unit, location of the conference room or meeting place, medication room, clean and dirty utility room, location of supplies and linen will help students to move around more efficiently in their environment and decrease the amount of time you spend redirecting them in the future. We also recommend that you provide a packet of informational items about the clinical unit, your "rules", information about assignments and the agency's patient care and medication administration and policies.

---

**AUTHORS' TIP**

Make up a scavenger hunt for the first day of clinical. Create a list of places and things you want the students to find on the unit. You may be specific for things they will use on a regular basis such as bedpans and the blood pressure cuffs. This can lessen anxiety and allow them to find their way around the unit.

---

As mentioned in Chapter Two, your students may need to receive EMR documentation system training or completion of competency modules on that first day of clinical. If so, be sure to weave this time into your first day or early in the rotation so students will possess documentation efficiency.

The students' level of experience will influence the amount of detail and time that you need to spend on EMR training. Students at the beginning of a nursing program are very anxious and unfamiliar with the routine on a nursing unit. Advanced students require less time to acclimate themselves, for they are familiar with the expectations of providing patient care. In either scenario do not expect to accomplish much patient care on the first day. You will discover that your orientation is time well spent!

We suggest that Form 4A the Pre-Clinical Student Self Reflection assignment be completed by every student in your group to provide you with information about themselves and their current knowledge. This can be revisited at the end of the clinical rotation, using the Post-Clinical Student Self Reflection (Form 4B) to summarize their growth, strengths and weaknesses and identify areas to focus on next semester. Providing your students with a list, agenda, or outline of what a typical clinical day looks like will help them stay on task and make your job easier. Refer to the Appendix: Example 4C – Typical Clinical Day provides a completed agenda for a structured clinical day. Form 4C is blank for you to create your own "typical" clinical day.

Remind students during their orientation, and at regular intervals, that paper documents containing patient information is protected by the HIPAA rules. As an added safety habit, routinely collect sensitive or private information from students at the end of the clinical day to ensure does it not leave the hospital and dispose of it properly. Students value this information as they use data to complete assignments such as care plans, but they must not take it home with them.

## DETERMINING STUDENT NURSE ASSIGNMENTS

As the instructor you should be prepared to arrive on the nursing unit at least an hour or more ahead of the students to make their assignment. It is a great strategy to develop a relationship with staff on the previous shift. This will afford you the necessary time and resources to ask them for input on the patient assignments. It also allows you an opportunity to view the medications that the patients will receive during your clinical day, and briefly review any patient conditions and diagnoses to assist you with selecting the best patient care assignment to meet the learning outcomes for the students.

### KNOW YOUR STUDENTS AND THE NURSING UNIT

Prior to making the actual clinical assignments you need to answer a few questions: What is the nursing level of the students? Are they fundamental level students at the beginning of the program, or do you have upper level nursing students whose knowledge base and skill set is more advanced? If the students have never worked in a hospital and this is their first clinical, you may want to partner the students with an unlicensed assistive personnel (UAP) to make the experience less stressful. Some institutions may refer to this staff member as a nursing assistant (NA), or patient care technician (PCT). Working with a partner eases them into the hospital setting.

In the beginning of a new clinical rotation, do not trust anyone but yourself. Both the students and the staff must earn your trust. Students generally start with a similar level of knowledge of nursing practice. During your observation of student performance, you will begin to note their progress and gain confidence in their abilities. Although you must remain aware of their activities, with time, they can work more independently. This is part of your evaluation of their progression and outcome attainment.

You already know that professional nurses possess their own philosophy and values. You will quickly identify nurses who are better role models for your students and which nurses may be not suited to work with a student. You will quickly know who the nurses are that are interested in education and happy to assist the students with their learning and sharing feedback with you. Do not expect the nurses on the unit to teach or observe skills you have not seen the student perform; you must assess the student yourself!

Assess the type of nursing unit your clinical group is assigned to. What is the specialty and patient acuity level? This will identify typical medications, treatments and possibly activity restrictions of the patients. Form 4D, Patient Care Type, can assist you with tracking students' assignments and guide you to vary the clinical experiences encounter each clinical day. Fill out the form with your students' names and the different diagnoses of the typical patients for the assigned clinical unit. See Example 4D in the Appendix for guidance.

### HOW TO CHOOSE PATIENTS

Nursing staff may assist you in assigning the best patients. They can advise you of patients that have interesting treatments or are in isolation. Avoid assigning a student to a patient with complex social or family issues. Do not assign patients that will be leaving the unit for an extended period, who are in respiratory isolation requiring an N95 mask, or an actively dying patient, unless death and dying are part of the course objectives.

Although it is exciting to assign patients with numerous interesting diagnoses and treatments, recognize that this may be overwhelming for you since you will likely oversee each of those treatments, depending on the knowledge level of your students. Medication administration, managing the tube feeding for patients with a gastrostomy tube, changing surgical dressings and monitoring chest tubes makes for a very interesting clinical day, but it can be a management nightmare for the instructor to observe each student and safely assess their clinical skill performance.

While determining the daily assignments, review each Medication Administration Record (MAR) to decide which patients will be assigned to receive medication from the students. Refer to Chapter Six for detailed information on the medication administration process. Medication administration is stressful for students, and the instructor. A strategy for safely supervising a group of students with reduced stress is to assign students alternate days to administer medications. If you choose to do this, the students who are not giving medications can benefit from assessing and providing total care to two or more of their patients. This will focus learning on disease processes and treatments. It is important to teach nursing students that medication administration is not the sole aspect of nursing care. This also provides them the opportunity to explore and seek other knowledge about laboratory results, disease processes, and the rationale for nursing care that accompanies it.

Form 4F, Clinical Activity and Assignment Calendar, can help you organize the rotation of medication administration and can be used to keep track of patient assignments or off unit experiences. See Example 4F in the Appendix to illustrate its use. Completed by you ahead of time and provided to the students it can prepare them for what they will be doing every clinical day. When a copy is provided to each student it keeps everyone organized.

### CONSIDER THE NURSES' ASSIGNMENT

Review the unit's nursing assignments and divide your students as evenly as possible among the nurses. Even though you will be supervising the students, the clinical nurses still maintain responsibility for patient care and will be communicating and working closely with the student. Avoid assigning any nurse more than two students if possible. Provide the clinical nurses with Form 4E, Student Assignments so they are informed of the student nurses' patient care assignments and the care that they will be providing. Clearly note on the assignment sheet if a student is administering medications for their assigned patients.

### CHANGING A STUDENT ASSIGNMENT

Sometimes a student assignment may have to be changed. Inform all relevant staff of the new assignment to assure care will be provided. Situations include: A patient's condition becomes critical and they are transferred to a higher level of care, or when a patient refuses to allow a student to care for them. The patient will usually agree to participate in most instances when you talk to them and reinforce that the student is working with the assigned nurse and the instructor, who is also a nurse. However, if the refusal remains, you must honor their wishes and reassign the student.

## THE STUDENTS' ARRIVAL TO CLINICAL

Students should be informed of the time to arrive on the nursing unit and where you will be meeting. The level of the students will determine your need to conduct a formal pre-conference meeting to review medical abbreviations and diagnoses for students near the beginning of their nursing program. More advanced students may not require a pre-conference. When students arrive to clinical, provide them with their patient assignment(s), any pertinent information and whether they are passing medications that day. Inform the students which nurse(s), and UAP(s) that they will be working with.

### *ORGANIZING YOUR STUDENTS AND THEIR PATIENTS*

Inform students of various resources available for them to gather information about their assigned patients before they obtain verbal report. The medical record, a kardex, a unit report sheet or other agency specific resources may be used. Emphasize to the students that copying of any of these documents is prohibited due to privacy regulations. While the students are obtaining the report from their nurses, they should clearly communicate treatments and medications they will be providing to patients.

This time is also your chance to sit down and finish filling out forms that you will carry with you on the unit. Form 4G, Patient Information Chart, will provide you with patient information. Example 4G in the Appendix is filled out for you with two sample patients who are referenced throughout this book. This chart will contain information about the patients from the medical record, the nursing staff and your student. Patient protected information should not be included. Other important data to include is patient code status, isolation precautions and admitting diagnosis.

If possible, it is very helpful to have a patient assignment list which includes the patient's full name, room number, and hospital medical record number printed from the EMR. This can also be used as a guide to identify the patients when you are in the room with the students. Discard at the end of the clinical day along with any other protected information you collect from the students.

### FACILITATING COMMUNICATION

As the clinical day progresses on the nursing unit, continually check with your students to assess any changes that may have occurred in a patient's condition, medication orders, or treatments.

A nursing unit may use agency provided phones, or other means, for communication between all staff. If possible, obtain a phone if available, although this may not always be feasible. You may also use your personal cell phone if agency policy permits so students may reach you directly when they need your assistance. The ability to contact you swiftly prevents them spending time trying to locate you. Students should also know where to locate the phone numbers of their nurse and UAP so they can readily contact them when needed.

### FACILITATING THE LEARNING PROCESS

As you oversee your students providing their patient care, documenting everything is imperative. Example 4H, the Student Clinical Day Progress Report in the Appendix, is a sample illustrating two student patient assignments. It demonstrates a convenient way of tracking each student's daily progress of completing documentation, treatments and medication administration for their assigned patients. Using the Student Clinical Day Progress Report (Form 4H) you may adapt this form to fit your clinical experience by designating the column headings to correlate with the documentation and skills that your students will be performing. The last column is for brief anecdotal notes about student performance. To assure compliance with HIPAA, only write the patient's initials, age and room number on the form. This will provide you with enough information to reference the correct patient when reviewing any subsequent written assignments you may be grading.

Form 4H also permits you to quickly note the students who have not completed assigned tasks. When you note the time documentation was completed on this form, it can be a measure of their weekly progress. The form is also a helpful tool to identify skills that students have not yet had an opportunity to experience.

Make rounds on your students to verify that they are beginning their assessments, looking up the medications they will administer, and providing patient care. Meet with each student to see if they received anything in the handoff report you need to know about or that requires clarification. This includes medication order changes, new physician orders, information or any special instructions including patient treatments.

Your clinical day will consist of overseeing medication administration, reviewing documentation and observing any procedures students perform on their patients to validate their technical skill and rationale for the treatment. A significant amount of time will also be spent observing student communication. Students will learn the importance of fostering effective communication between the assigned patients, significant others, the nursing staff and you.

---

**AUTHORS' TIP**

When students are in their first rotation and focusing on basic patient care, if they are caught up, and their patient is going to x-ray, or other nonsurgical or endoscopic procedures, allow the student to go with them. Check with the department first, but most will allow students to accompany their patient.

If a patient you have assigned to your student has an interesting wound, drainage tube, or a dialysis shunt, inquire if the patient would mind if other students may view it. Most patients are willing to allow this.

---

### STUDENT DOCUMENTATION

Students should be informed of the patient care documentation they are responsible for during their shift. This may include physical assessment, safety documentation, vital signs, intake and output and narrative chart entries.

Plan for available time between medication administration and observing skills to review their documentation. If a student needs to write a narrative note, we suggest a written draft be required to check grammar, spelling and accuracy prior to entering it into the medical record. All documentation will need to be reviewed and co-signed by you, and before the students leave for the day. Ongoing review of the documentation will assure you stay current, and it is completed, at the end of the clinical day. Refer to Chapter Six for more about medication administration documentation.

### PROVIDING SAFE PATIENT CARE

Encourage teamwork among the students so they can care for their patients safely and complete their work on time. Encourage the students to continually be sure their patients are safe, with side rails up, bed in lowest position, call button within reach, and the room is free of barriers to prevent falls. To facilitate continuity of care, teach your students the proper way to report off to the nursing staff when leaving for break and at the end of the clinical day.

As your students reach higher levels in the nursing program their clinical experience will also increase in complexity. Students will be caring for more than one patient and providing more intricate nursing skills. A strategy to promote safety and to decrease your responsibility of overseeing eight to ten students directly is to arrange for alternative experiences and assignments as discussed in Chapter Seven.

### TIME MANAGEMENT

Teaching personal time management skills is essential for students. Teach and role model the concepts of teamwork, prioritization and organization of their work load. Planning a break and meal time into a student's day is one of the most important lessons you can teach. Most nurses work hard, believe they must accomplish everything, and frequently do not allow themselves time to take a break or eat a meal. Do not forget to take a break yourself! Oversight of eight to ten students is exhausting.

### POST-CONFERENCE

Post-conference is a vital conclusion to the clinical day. Ideally it should take place in a private conference room away from staff, patients and visitors. At a minimum it should be 60 to

90 minutes. It is during this conference the students get to share or "debrief" their experiences. Discussions may include a patient's diagnosis and interesting information students learned during their encounters. A HIPAA violation can be prevented when patient privacy is stressed, and each student is allowed the opportunity to share their day in a secluded area. No matter how many clinical days a nursing student has completed they always need to share their experiences with others. This is also the opportunity for you to collect and destroy any protected patient information.

Allow students to share their encounters, both positive and negative, during confidential post-conferences. Any difficult moments students experienced with nursing staff may be discussed at this time. Observations of questionable nursing practice may also be mentioned. This information may later be relayed to a nurse manager by you, but always encourage students to feel safe sharing. Post-conference needs to be viewed by the students as a safe place to express their feelings about what happened during the clinical day. It is impossible to determine prior experiences a student brings to clinical that may trigger emotions.

## POST-CONFERENCE IDEAS

Full time faculty can provide information and ideas to guide you. Many times, the type of clinical day that was experienced will direct the conversation. Everyone participates in post-conference and is provided with the opportunity to ask and answer questions from both the instructor and their peers. Students can provide a patient "problem" or nursing diagnosis for their patient. Students may be assigned to report about a drug they administered or share information they researched during the clinical day. Instructor observations of the group's organizational and time management skills may be discussed, and recommendations for improvement provided. The post-conference is a continuation of the clinical learning experience. Pertinent theory course information or a scholarly journal article related to the patient population can be a focus of post-conference. Relevant pathophysiology or math calculations can be reviewed as needed. Quizzing or other games may assist students to better understand disease process and correlate it to the patient population.

If a student has participated in an alternative assignment, or an off-unit observation, they can share their experiences. Students may work on any clinical assignments or utilize the hospital library to complete their concept maps and care plan assignments as a group. Some clinical rotations involve student presentations on various topics. Post-conference is a perfect time for any of these examples to occur.

### DISCUSSION OF ERRORS

Student errors may be discussed, but only as a learning opportunity for the group. Minor mishaps such as pulling the tubing out of the intravenous bag before turning it upside down can help peers avoid the same mistake and can be humorous if no harm occurred. It is advisable these discussions be approached in a generic manner so that students are not singled out or embarrassed in front of their peers. Students may be willing share to their mistake with their peers on their own, however you must be aware of the possibility of a Family Educational Rights and Privacy Act (FERPA) violation. Student records and educational rights are protected in higher education in the same way as patients are with the HIPAA. If an individual student's performance did not meet the expected standards do not discuss this with the group. This is reserved for a private meeting.

## INSTRUCTOR'S CLINICAL DOCUMENTATION OF STUDENT PERFORMANCE

The end of the clinical day is your opportunity for a documentation session. Wrap up your day by sitting down and reflecting how it went. This is the time to review your students' performance. You may need to make more anecdotal notes that will serve as your record of situations that occurred at clinical. They could be as minor as "all students need to be more organized to complete their assignments on time", to the more specific "student A needs another chance to improve the administration of insulin". If students are progressing well, you may choose not to make any notes on a day.

You must document a more comprehensive narrative of an occurrence that deems further observation of a student's progress. This is extremely important in the event a remediation is needed or a failure occurs. Use of our tools will support your evaluation of student performance that did not meet the minimum requirements for success. See Chapter Nine for further discussion regarding the remediation process and a template to assist you with evaluating student progress.

Along with this reflection process it is helpful to make a note about the students' participation on Form 4I, Skills Checklist. This form will be helpful on the next clinical day when making assignments and identifies students who need a specific experience. This is an easy way to ascertain all students are getting a variety of learning opportunities. This also prevents the same student from inadvertently get all, or no, skills opportunity. Refer to Example 4I, Skills Checklist, in the Appendix to guide you with its use.

You are making assignments for your students on a busy medical-surgical unit. Today you have seven students on the unit and one student in the operating room. The nurses tell you there are several good learning opportunities, including post-operative patients whose care might include dressing changes, pain medications or discharge instructions. This is your third week of clinical, so you refer to your list of student experiences from the previous weeks to assist you in making assignments.

So many great learning opportunities. . . . how do you choose?

**First you might want to make a list like this:**

- Patient 1– post-op day one, new colostomy, four oral medications, one antibiotic and intravenous (IV) fluids
- Patient 2 – post-op day one, colostomy revision (patient self-sufficient with ostomy care) five oral medications, one IV antibiotic
- Patient 3 – post-op day two, major abdominal surgery with epidural pain pump and nasogastric tube (NGT), two oral medications, three IV antibiotics, and primary IV fluid monitoring
- Patient 4 – bowel obstruction with NGT, IV fluids and five oral medications
- Patient 5 – transurethral prostate resections (TURP) going home, needs teaching, four oral medications
- Patient 6 – TURP going home, needs teaching, 10 oral medications
- Patient 7 – abdominal wound infection, extensive dressing change, four oral medications, two IV antibiotics
- Patient 8 – exacerbation of Crohn's disease, total parenal

nutrition (TPN) via a central line, three oral medications and IV fluids
- Patient 9 – diverticulitis, IV antibiotics, four oral medications
- Patient 10 – post-op day three, abdominal surgery, 10 oral medications, IV fluid monitoring
- Patient 11 – pancreatitis, history of alcoholism (ETOH) pain medications, IV fluid monitoring, four oral medications

**Next, look over your student list and decide how to assign them**. For example: three of the students never had an ostomy patient, two students never had a patient with an NGT, one student needs a challenge today and Patient 3 might be a good assignment. Continue referring to your student clinical needs list and make the assignments that will provide the best learning opportunities.

Remember you will need to be present when your students administer medications, perform dressing changes, and provide patient teaching to their patients, particularly the TURP patients. You will also follow up on the students who have patients with NGTs, TPN and the epidural to provide specific teaching-learning opportunities. Therefore, choosing the patients requires that you plan out your day ahead of time to assure your ability for effective management of the students' assignments.

Consider which students will administer medications and review the medication profile of the patients you wish to assign. Referring to the list above will assist you in providing a great clinical day that does not overwhelm either the students or you. If your students can care for two patients, choose extra patients for those students not administering medications. Notice that one of the TURP patients has 10 oral medications.

If you want to assign this patient do not have the student give medications, or just assign one TURP. Both patients may require too much of your time and keep you from monitoring the other students in your group effectively.

The nursing staff can assist in observing your students. However, remember that you are responsible for observing and gathering information about your student's clinical performance to attest to their clinical competency. Choose assignments carefully, since you cannot be everywhere at once!

The development of critical thinking

# Five

We must include a discussion about critical thinking. Much has been published, discussed, and examined about its importance in nursing education. As a new educator you may wish to spend time reviewing these resources.

Many nursing students believe academic success, demonstrated by a high-grade point average, are guarantees for the successful completion of a nursing program. Students who are "book smart" are not always the best bedside nurses. Intellectual ability, although obviously necessary to be a nurse, must be accompanied by skills such as the ability to critically think using higher order anticipatory and problem solving strategies. Manual dexterity and an aptitude for interpersonal communication are also necessary attributes to become a successful nurse.

Your success as a nurse and your decision to pursue the role of a clinical instructor indicates that you possess strong critical thinking skills and recognize their influence on a student nurse. The nursing process is the way your students will learn to create a plan for their assigned patients. You will guide them through deciding on a nursing diagnosis, identify outcomes, plan interventions and evaluate the plan. Nursing diagnosis, interventions, and rationale for care are what nursing education and practice own: It is the "why" of what we do versus just "completing a task".

Clinical assignments may already be developed using a nursing theory as the framework. Assignments may include: Journaling, reflective papers, care plans and concept maps about an assigned patient and health care team interactions. These assignments, along with clinical observation and interaction provides you with some measurable evidence of a student's critical thinking. Discussions during your pre- or post-conference time may be another means to observe this skill. The course syllabus will determine what the expectations are for clinical assignments.

## THE CONCEPT MAP CARE PLAN

You may not be familiar with using a concept map care plan. It is an organizational tool that provides the opportunity for a student to demonstrate their use of the nursing process related to their assigned patient. It should include a nursing diagnosis, detailed explanation of their goals and plan of care for their patient. Other items that may be reported include an analysis of laboratory and diagnostic findings and relationships to the diagnosis. Some nursing schools provide templates for students to follow. Students are provided with education on construction of these maps along with guidelines about the formation and use of the nursing process. Your lead faculty member may provide you with a format and example, so you can learn how to guide your students and adequately assess their critical thinking. Form 5A, the Concept Map Template, can be used if you are not provided with one. Example 5A, Concept Map, found in the Appendix, illustrates how a student may use this tool to demonstrate their "thinking" surrounding nursing care for the patient Mrs. M. who will be presented in Scenario 5-1 further in this chapter. A concept map should lead to detail assessment findings and logical, appropriate patient care interventions.

Most nursing schools require students to purchase a nursing diagnosis textbook. Obtaining your own copy will assist you immensely when it comes time to evaluate and grade these assignments.

## GRADING CLINICAL ASSIGNMENTS

A substantial responsibility as a clinical instructor is reading, reviewing and grading clinical assignments and care maps. This CANNOT be done during clinical time. New clinical faculty may not be fully aware of this responsibility. Grading student assignments is part of your commitment to clinical teaching and is time consuming, but guidance from your lead faculty member can be invaluable and may provide tools that will walk you through a written assignment review that may decrease grading time.

## NURTURING CRITICAL THINKING IN YOUR STUDENTS

Although clinical assignments and exercises are very useful, critical thinking and the measurement of it remains elusive. The goal is to help student nurses recognize the real-world scenarios that nurses face deciding on interventions to attain the best outcome for their patients. Your role is to guide your students to utilize critical thinking in every aspect of their nursing care and to make the connections between what they write on their care plan and the actual nursing interventions they provide.

You need to make use of every teachable moment that occurs in a clinical day. This is the exciting part of clinical teaching. When you see the recognition on a student's face when their learning meets reality and they have an "Aha" moment; it can be very rewarding. When students see that you are excited about their learning they too become excited and eager to put their theoretical learning into practice.

Problem based learning and thinking is a strategy that a clinical instructor can use to help a student plan for the unexpected needs of a patient, the "what ifs". The clinical instructor working with a student nurse has an excellent opportunity to coach a student through such situations, usually one-on-one. From our experience, prompting students using open-ended questions will enhance the development of a student's problem-solving skills. The goal is that these steps become habitual and increase in complexity as exposure to more clinical situations occur. Many times, students know the answer or solution, but need your guidance to feel confident in their knowledge. By asking the right questions students can be coached to self-realization that they really do know how to proceed in a situation. Many researchers have published information about critical thinking that you may wish to review and integrate into your teaching.

Encourage your students to ask questions about their patient, care, and diagnosis but avoid providing immediate answers. Instead direct them to find the answer themselves. For example: A student inquires if they should reconnect their patient's nasogastric tube (NGT) to suction. Easy answer is to "check with the nurse". The better answer to pose is "why do you think the NGT is disconnected?" When you respond to students in a non-threatening and encouraging way they will seek answers independently to challenge their thinking and enhance learning.

### CRITICAL THINKING EXAMPLES

Below are examples of clinical scenarios and some suggestions for probing questions that will help you guide students through a nursing care critical thinking exercise. These patients are referred to in Chapter Four and are referred to on the clinical forms and examples mentioned.

During a first medical-surgical rotation you have assigned to a student Mrs. M., a widowed 76-year-old female patient admitted with the diagnosis of transient ischemic attack (TIA). The patient also has a history of Type 2 diabetes, hypertension, and breast cancer with subsequent right radical mastectomy at age 65. The student has received report from the assigned nurse and is provided with additional information.

0600 Assessment:

- Alert and oriented x 2–3, occasional confusion about being in the hospital
- BP 170/94, Pulse – 68 Respirations – 20 per minute, $PaO_2$–95% on room air
- 0600 Fasting blood sugar (FBS) – 206
- Activity: bathroom privileges with assistance, fall risk, bed alarm
- Scheduled diagnostics: Head computed tomography (CT) no contrast
- Labs: FBS, and blood sugar (BS) every 6 hours with sliding scale coverage of regular insulin; complete blood count (CBC) and electrolytes daily
- Medications that are ordered include: Metformin, Lisinopril, and Tamoxifen

Formulate questions that will validate that the student can devise a plan of care integrating acquired knowledge from theory. Some examples follow.

*What are your concerns related to the information you were given during the shift report that will impact the care you provide to your patient?*

Ideally the student will mention the past medical history and how it may have influenced the current situation for the patient. They should discuss these findings: Altered mental status, safety concerns, elevated blood pressure, including restrictions about the use of the arm on the mastectomy side, discussion about how blood pressure relates to the current diagnosis, the prescribed medications, and the elevated glucose level.

During the discussion about each concern you have an opportunity to expound on multiple areas of the student's knowledge, providing an excellent opportunity for an evaluation moment with the student. Acknowledging their level of understanding of the assessment data, and asking probing questions to get a desirable answer, requires participation by the student. If you note that a student requires an extensive amount of prompting about information that they should be familiar with, this may require further remediation. This will be discussed later but must be anecdotally documented by you as soon as possible.

Here are a few more relevant questions you can pose to the student:

*What is your priority goal for the care of this patient during your shift?*

*What interventions will you implement to assure the patient's safety?*

*What do you note about the vital sign and laboratory trends for this patient over the past 24 hours?*

*What further actions related to these findings may be necessary for you to take? Why?*

*After a quick overview of the record, how will you plan for medication administration for this patient?*

*What other medical history will impact the care you will be providing to this patient?*

Here is another example of a teachable moment utilizing critical thinking:

## SCENARIO 5-2: MR. R.

A nursing student inquired why their patient, Mr. R., was receiving an antibiotic and antiviral drug when they could not find any history of infections in his chart. The instructor asked the student about the patient's diagnosis. The student stated "leukemia". Through a series of probing questions, the student learned that it was the chemotherapy that put the patient at risk for infections when the white blood cell count dropped. The student was sent to look up the chemotherapy since they were not administering it. They subsequently learned about the Nadir–the time when the counts are the lowest–and prophylactic drug therapy. The student shared what they learned through this process in the post-conference.

Teaching strategies such as these help the student internalize the learning. They must assess learned concepts, build on that knowledge, look up information, and then teach their peers what they learned from the experience. In Scenario 5-2, it would have been much simpler for the instructor to just answer the question, but the student gained much more knowledge this way.

Similarly, whenever a student must perform a hands-on procedure or skill, prior to entering the patient room ask them to not only explain and demonstrate to you, if possible, what they are about to do, but also ask them to verbalize the rationale for completing it and describe any teaching they will need to provide to the patient. Again, this illustrates they know and understand what they are doing, why they are doing it, and it builds student confidence.

# Six

Nursing students only acquire confidence for the important skill of medication administration by performing it on live human beings. You are the guardian of both the patient and the student during this process. As the licensed professional the burden of responsibility falls onto you to protect the patient and assure safe practice occurs. As an educator your goal is to teach students the significant responsibility they are assuming and establish processes they can carry into their own practice.

Preparing ahead and using some of the strategies that we are suggesting, can make this aspect of your role less intimidating. As you are teaching medication administration to nursing students we are confident you may devise your own "system". We have provided forms to guide, organize, and assist you while ensuring medications are administered to patients by the student safely, and timely. We suggest avoiding assigning patients who will receive multiple medications during a shift for it will quickly become time consuming and make you unavailable to the remaining students.

### PRE-CLINICAL PREPARATION

It is extremely important to acquaint yourself with the medication administration processes and documentation procedures during your meeting with the nurse manager. Arranging time on the nursing unit prior to clinical to observe this activity is important. You will want to learn about the electronic medication dispensing system, if used, and how medications are documented when given. Ask about agency medication policies that exist. These actions will prepare you to function in your role as a clinical instructor more confidently when you are working with students.

The medication rooms in some agencies may only be accessed with an identification badge or other security measures. You will need to obtain approval for your access. While overseeing medication administration on the nursing unit, follow the procedures students are currently being taught versus what you may have learned decades ago. Visit the nursing skills laboratory to witness students practicing medication administration. This will provide to you up to date evidence-based information and techniques. Also, if you are unfamiliar with the intravenous pumps or other medication devices being used on the nursing unit, seek help to learn how to operate them.

You will want to devise a system to document your students' schedule for medication administration to aid in your organization. Form 6A, Medication Administration Tracking Record will help with this task. We have also provided Example 6A in the Appendix as a sample of how this form may be used for two students administering medications.

### YOUR SAFE PRACTICE

As an experienced nurse we know it may be tempting to devise ways to save time during the busy clinical day. Medication administration is a time-consuming task when working with student nurses and requires patience. Remember you are thinking with an experienced practitioner's mind who has administered medications to hundreds or thousands of patients. Now, you have committed to teach and mentor future nurses who do not possess your knowledge.

Unfortunately, you may encounter nurses who override the electronic medication dispensing systems. These actions disregard policy and contribute to an unsafe culture of shortcuts. An example: A second nurse, who does not want to wait her turn for the dispensing machine, reaches into an open drawer to retrieve a dose of a medication while another nurse is removing medications for their patient. The second nurse could easily make an error and retrieve a wrong dose. This scenario also bypasses the safeguards of double-checking the patient's medication profile, including the "right" patient, "right" medication, "right" dose. Similar appearances of some drug packaging, and the haste of the second nurse, might result in a dangerous error. Role modeling patience and methodical practice to your students will prevent such mistakes from occurring.

### FLEXIBILITY REQUIRED

Oversight of multiple nursing students is hard work, and medication administration is time consuming if it is to be accomplished safely. Plan on experiencing days when you cannot have all students administer medications. Other days it may require that you ask the assigned nurse to do it to avoid delays. We guarantee this will happen, and although you may feel it is a failure on your part, it is not. Patient care cannot be delayed. Situations on the nursing unit can change rapidly and do not always afford you the opportunity to re-prioritize patient care goals. Compare this to your own practice when an emergency or unexpected task had to be handled first. If a patient had chest pain and it became an emergency code situation, did your colleagues quickly intervene without question to provide care and medications for your other patients? Of course, they did!

If you cannot provide a medication administration experience for a student have them observe a nurse doing it. This can still be a valuable learning opportunity for the student. Patients assigned to student nurses who request medications for pain control may need to be deferred to the nurse if you predict a delay in administration. Students should recognize this as a priority, and that timely pain relief must be provided. Encourage the student to accompany the nurse, so they may witness how controlled substances are retrieved and a pain assessment on the patient is documented. If a student witnesses questionable or unsafe practice while accompanying a nurse administering medications, this is an educational opportunity to discuss with the clinical group privately in post-conference.

## GUIDING THE MEDICATION ADMINISTRATION SEQUENCE

The actual administration of a medication to a patient and documentation on the medication MAR by a nursing student is a small part of the whole process. Student preparation is the key to assure that safety is maintained, while allowing them to critically think about the task at hand. A template for medication preparation for student use is provided in Form 6B, Student Medication Preparation. This will provide structure and help students provide organized information about the medications they will be giving, which supports your evaluation of their competence. Example 6B, found in the Appendix, is filled out with Mrs. M.'s medications.

The following is a sequence for verifying students' knowledge and preparation of medication administration and supervising the actual skill.

- *Ask the student why the patient is receiving the ordered medication and any relevant associated data.*

Students must be allotted time to look up the medications they will be administering. They should be able to verbalize the admitting diagnosis and any pathophysioloy that provides rationale for each medication they will administer. Prompts from you as the instructor using probing questions to assess knowledge may include:

- *Is the patient diabetic? Is there a history of cardiac disease? Are they postoperative?*
- *Does the patient have any allergies?*
- *What is the administration route?*
- *Can the patient swallow?*
- *What classification of medication is this?*
- *Is a safe dose ordered?*
- *Are there assessments that must be performed or reviewed? Current vital signs and significant lab results?*
- *Any side effects of concern?*
- *When was the last dose given?*

Verify that the current medication dose about to given has not been administered earlier by the nurse. This is another reason for you to make frequent rounds and practice open communication with the nurses. Always double-check time frames for "as needed" (PRN) medications, to determine when they were last administered. If a student cannot verbalize these facts or confidently answer questions you must not allow them to administer medications. Send the student to investigate the answers, gain further information and report back to you so they may complete the task. A student, who views "giving a pill" as only that, requires much more coaching and evaluation. If a student can demonstrate the link from a patient's diagnosis, pathophysiology of a disease, and medical history to an ordered medication with minimal prompts, you may proceed to the next step. Refer to Chapter Five for more on the critical thinking discussion if needed.

- *Allow the student time to examine the medication, obtain equipment if needed, and discuss the administration technique*

There are multiple resources in drug handbooks and the internet that may be utilized. Discussion surrounding student understanding about the various forms of medication along with review of techniques for administration must occur prior to entering a patient room. Students may need time to locate tubing, syringes and injection needles. Allow for this time; it will become shorter as their exposure to these experiences recurs. Intravenous calculations must also be completed before attempting to program an infusion pump. Calculators are a must!

- *You and the student must appear confident when administering medications to a patient, or a patient may refuse to allow the action.*

Alert students that patients or significant others are watching their actions more closely than you are, and they will quickly detect doubt or uncertainty if hesitation occurs. If the student stumbles, you must gracefully step in to maintain the patient and significant others' confidence and possibly completing the task.

- *Never send a student to administer medications alone.*

No shortcuts are allowed during this part of the teaching process! Most agencies require that an instructor cosign medication administration as soon as a student documents it. You must witness the student's performance, accuracy and assure that they follow the rights of medication administration. Fatal mistakes can occur if a student is not competent and you are not present to prevent an error. As the instructor, your role is to evaluate the student's performance. When a student repeatedly does not check the wristband of a confused patient, despite reminders and remediation, they ultimately may fail clinical. Without instructor observation, this behavior could continue and a tragic medication error could occur now, or in the future.

- Debrief the student after the medication administration encounter.

If the encounter was successful, offer praise immediately to solidify the student's learning experience and increase their confidence. Students that perceive success will strive to repeat their behavior in future instances of medication administration. If a student performed poorly, a private discussion with documentation of the performance deficiency must occur on the same day. Refer to Form 4H, Student Clinical Day Progress Report which has a place to quickly make a notation about medication administration performance. Example 4H in the Appendix illustrates this documentation. A plan for remediation must be created for the student with poor performance. The school's nursing skills laboratory can assure that due process and opportunity for improvement is provided. A student should not participate in medication administration until a remediation has satisfactorily been concluded. Refer to your program's policy and abide by it. Chapter Nine will provide more detail about remediation. Repeated episodes of poor student performance during medication administration will result in a clinical failure.

- Documentation on the patient's medical record must immediately occur after the medication has been administered.

If a medication is not administered as the result of a patient refusal or the vital signs or laboratory values are not within safe parameters, the nurse must be notified. If a medication must be rescheduled for a later time it is recommended that the nurse complete that task, so it is entered correctly on the MAR.

- If students will be administering newly ordered medications, coordinate this with the nurse so missed doses or double dosing do not occur.
- If a patient's medications are missing or the student has a question about compatibility, allow the student to call the pharmacy department themselves.

This action fosters interdisciplinary collaboration and strengthens professional communication skills. Instruct the student to not only identify the patient but also to identify themselves as a student nurse when initiating this communication.

> ### AUTHORS' TIP
>
> Give medications last to patients who need their drugs crushed or dispensed via gastronomy and feeding tubes. This will lessen your sense of urgency about being timely with administration since this task is time-consuming, but a great learning experience.

## STUDENT MEDICATION ERRORS AND OTHER INCIDENTS

Student medication errors must be handled immediately. Patient safety is of utmost importance. First assess the patient. Inform the patient's nurse who will then notify the attending physician of the error. Documentation of the circumstances should be completed per agency policy and nursing program policy on the appropriate forms. The student must be interviewed, and detailed information gathered about how the error transpired. Continued assessment of the patient must also occur to observe for any negative consequences. These occurrences should be handled as a teaching and learning experience for a student and thoroughly documented by you. Document an anecdotal note for your own records in the event follow up information is needed by the agency. Refer to Chapter Four for documenting this anecdotal note, which will be used for student evaluation purposes.

Reinforce to students the importance of continuously focusing on the "rights" of medication administration to prevent errors. Not every agency will have electronic medication dispensing systems. There is a greater risk of administering medications to the wrong patient when nursing students are only exposed to sophisticated electronic medication dispensing systems. Nursing programs also teach manual methods. Technology does not remove human error in any setting and they must develop habits that ensure safety to the patient.

Although education about preventing exposure is provided in nursing skills laboratories a student is still at risk for injury while in a clinical setting. A needle stick or exposure to body fluids is always a possibility. If this occurs, the nursing school must be notified, and relevant documentation completed. It may be required that the student follow up with a physician. Some nursing schools may require participating students to carry health insurance for this reason. Contact your lead faculty member to guide you in these instances.

## SCENARIO 6-1 STUDENT MEDICATION ADMINISTRATION SCENARIO

Your student, Tim, states he is ready to give medication to his patient. You follow the guidelines outlined in the medication administration process. Tim answers all your questions correctly and is well prepared. He knows all about his patient's condition and medical history. He also correctly provides the current glucose result and vital signs. Tim obtains the medications from the dispensing machine, selecting all the correct drugs from the MAR and pulling them out of the compartments.

Tim begins to prepare to draw up the insulin dosage. He grabs a TB syringe instead of the correct insulin syringe. You step in and inquire if he has the correct supplies. He looks flustered.

- Ask him "How is the dose written in the order?"
- Tim replies "4 units".
- Ask Tim, "Show me where the 4 unit mark is on the syringe?"

Tim immediately sees his mistake. Allow him to gather the correct syringe and draw up the insulin. Next, review the correct procedure by asking:

- "Where will you administer the injection?"
- "How will you dispose of the syringe?"
- "Does the patient need any teaching?"

If Tim is lacking in knowledge a second time use prompts to allow him time to correct any mistakes.

When Tim arrives at the bedside observe that he checks the name band and correctly verifies each medication with EMR. Be ready to step in if he starts to make an error.

Tim is getting ready to administer the insulin, but he is not wearing gloves. Call his name and remind him about the gloves. You may verbally remind him, grab a pair of gloves or show him your hands so he gets the message. The way you approach correcting a student depends on several variables: How quickly he is moving, how nervous the patient appears and your teaching style.

After the medications are administered, privately provide the student with a quick verbal critique:

- *"Good job but remember to grab gloves and tell the patient before you inject her."*

Before you proceed to the next student make a note on your Student Clinical Day Progress Report (Form 4H) about Tim's mistakes, and that he demonstrated fair technique while giving the injection.

# Seven

There may be alternative clinical experiences associated with your rotation. For example, having students to go to the operating room (OR) and follow a patient from pre-op, to the operating room, and then on to the post anesthesia care unit (PACU) is something that may occur during a medical-surgical rotation. Other times you are offered an opportunity for students to go to the emergency room or shadow a clinical nurse specialist. Or maybe you want to develop your own clinical assignment or activity for students to complete. Before you plan these, it is advisable to share your ideas and intent with the lead faculty member who coordinates the course you are teaching. They will determine if these activities can occur and be included in your overall performance evaluation of the student. These experiences also must align with the course objectives and student learning outcomes published in the syllabus. The alternative clinical experience or assignment is a way to decrease the number of students you must supervise directly and allow those remaining more of your time and attention. Reducing your assignment by one student can make a difference for you, especially on a busy nursing unit. It is also interesting for all students to experience different aspects of nursing.

## IDEAS FOR ALTERNATIVE CLINICAL ASSIGNMENTS AND EXPERIENCES

Ideas for alternative clinical experiences include: Shadowing a clinical nurse educator, a wound care nurse, a nurse manager, or by visiting a specialty center such a radiation oncology center or hemodialysis unit. Examples of alternative experiences that may not necessarily remove the student from the clinical unit but can be implemented by a clinical instructor include: Team leading, completion of a quality or safety audit, chart review, or researching a topic or procedure relevant to the nursing unit or a theory course learning outcome. Consider consulting with the nurse manager to identify unit initiatives where students may be able to assist.

### STUDENT ENGAGEMENT

When students participate in an alternative assignment there must be a defined written assignment associated with the experience. This focuses a student's learning and promotes their engagement. Assignments need to be meaningful and add an additional dimension to patient care. Students must follow the rules set forth by the clinical agency, which may limit the amount of hands-on experience they can attain during their alternative experience. Some agencies require that the clinical instructor submit pre-defined learning outcomes for the student's experience. Attaching an assignment to this experience creates structure and provides evidence of accountability by the student, particularly when you are unable to be present. Example 7A, Alternative Experience: Visit to OR in the Appendix provides objectives for a student's experience in the OR and may be used if you need an assignment, or assistance with developing ideas for other areas.

## STUDENT TEAM LEADERS

For advanced clinical groups who have more clinical experience and are near the end of their program, generally in a final, or capstone course, a student may be assigned a team leadership role. Form 7B, Team Leader Responsibilities provides guidelines for the role. These may include: Obtaining a report from each student peer, rounding on the patients and obtaining updates about their progress. Form 7B may serve as a guide for students in this role.

Communicate to the designated student team leader that they may collaborate with other students to investigate and problem solve issues but must seek out the instructor or the staff nurse if major questions arise. The team leader may assist other students with patient care and treatments, researching medications and developing plans of care. The assigned student will provide you with a comprehensive summary report of the team's status at the end of the shift. Remember, however, you remain the licensed professional and responsible individual for the team assignment!

### *EVALUATING YOUR STUDENT TEAM LEADER*

When a student completes the team leader "day" you must evaluate their performance managing of a group of student nurses, who are their "staff", and patients. A discussion of successes and challenges of the experience should be included. Critique their reporting of information and discuss any issues that they noted. This will instill greater confidence in their abilities and sense of collaboration. A written review of their strengths and weaknesses from you will give them time to "self reflect" on their experience.

### SBAR

Team leading is also an opportunity for a student to implement the situation, background, assessment, recommendation framework (SBAR) developed by Leonard, Bonacum, and Graham (2004). This communication model was modified for health care encounters from a similar framework used by the United States Navy (Leonard, et al., 2004). It may be adapted by students to illustrate their organization and prioritization skills. You may wish to include SBAR in a post-conference discussion to refine your students' communication skills.

#### SAMPLE SBAR COMMUNICATION

Here is an example of a SBAR interaction related to Patient Scenario 5-1, Mrs. M., from Chapter Five:

S (Situation) "I am updating you about Mrs. M., a 76-year-old female admitted with a TIA last evening. I have noted a right sided facial droop that was not present when I assessed her at 0800 a.m. Her blood pressure is elevated 184/100, this is an increase from 0600 a.m. when it was 170/94."

B (Background) "Mrs. M. has a history of Type 2 diabetes, hypertension and breast cancer with a right radical mastectomy. She is on metformin, lisinopril, and tamoxifen and received her medications as ordered at 0900 a.m. She had a negative head computed tomography (CT) without contrast completed upon admission."

A (Assessment) "I am very concerned about these changes in her neurological status and believe she may be actively having a stroke."

R (Recommendation) "I am requesting that the patient be evaluated as soon as possible so other interventions may be ordered to rule out or confirm a stroke."

## QUALITY AND SAFETY AUDIT ACTIVITIES

As mentioned in Chapter One, schools of nursing refer to the QSEN model to guide the use of alternative assignments. An example of this is to have the students visit an assigned group of patients and complete a safety check list. The check list could be provided by the agency or developed by you. Visit the QSEN website (www.QSEN.org) and review recommended teaching strategies for clinical instruction for other ideas.

A quality and safety activity example would be to have a student observe the nurse perform a specific procedure or nursing intervention and investigate it independently. Examples include: The choice of various pain control measures, administration of chemotherapy on an oncology unit or chest tube maintenance on a thoracic unit. Subsequently they will research the procedure in the agency's policy manual and on the internet. Comparison of the policy, the reference, and the observation of the procedure being performed may provide a learning opportunity. Locating policy and procedures and how they relate to evidence-based literature assists a student with recognizing the importance of the use of research in nursing practice. Students may then review the medical record to determine how and where the procedures are documented. Findings may be submitted in writing or presented in post-conference.

## ALTERNATIVE ASSIGNMENTS FOR CLINICAL ABSENCES

Refer to the lead faculty for the course you that you are teaching to familiarize yourself with the policy for clinical absences and options. Some schools may allow an absence without consequence while others are specific about how clinical hours may be duplicated. Clinical requirements including mandatory orientation and the use of different EMR systems among agencies make it almost impossible for students to make up missed clinical time in another group or agency. Several options for a "make up day" may be available. We have included several ideas used by nursing programs.

### CASE STUDIES

Some nursing textbook publishers provide case studies that may be assigned to students as a make-up assignment. Students are required to create a plan of care and detail how they will execute their goals for the assigned patient, similar to decision making in the real clinical setting, although one-dimensional. These modules are designed to be lengthy and specific. Your full-time lead faculty member can guide you to this option if it exists.

### HUMAN PATIENT SIMULATION

Human patient simulation is gaining momentum in nursing programs as a way for students to gain valuable clinical experience and explore other learning opportunities using the simulation laboratory. Quality simulation scenarios are commercially available to assist nursing faculty with engaging students in life-like clinical situations. There are numerous topics and levels of difficulty to choose from. Scenarios can be manipulated to create harm to the "patient" to promote student learning without jeopardizing a human life. Your nursing program may offer a simulation experience as an option for a student to make up missed clinical time.

Numerous research has been published about the quality of simulation as an alternate to clinical days in a hospital. Since clinical sites in many regions are limited and more difficult to obtain, simulation is becoming a standard teaching modality in nursing education, and, in some cases, it is replacing the actual clinical experience. Explore if simulation is an option in the nursing program you are teaching for.

## REFERENCE

Leonard, M., Bonacum, S., & Graham, D. (2004). The human factor: The critical importance of effective teamwork and communication in providing safe care. *Quality and Safety in Health Care.* Oct; 13 Suppl 1: i85–i90. doi: 10.1136/qshc.2004.010033.

Diversity and inclusiveness

# Eight

Knowledge of diversity and inclusiveness is vital in health care. Your students will encounter situations where they will want to help a patient but are uncertain of the next move due to beliefs, practices or customs that may differ from theirs. Although efforts to increase diversity in the workforce continue, the nursing profession is predominantly comprised of white females (Buerhaus, Skinner, Auerbach, & Staiger, 2017). Recruitment efforts to acquire nursing students representative of the diverse populations seeking healthcare in the United States continues. In our experience, if patients and their caregiver share similar belief systems, the patient is more likely to comply to their prescribed care, experience less anxiety and recover more quickly.

## DIVERSITY AWARENESS

The patient population at the agency where you are teaching clinical usually reflects the cultural and ethnic composition of the surrounding community. When meeting the nurse manager at the agency for clinical orientation inquire about the cultural or religious diversity of the patient population. Review any agency statements or policies about diversity that may exist. Responding with confidence and sensitivity to situations students may encounter during the clinical experience improves their ability to provide successful patient care.

Review any information surrounding diversity that is included in nursing program curriculum before the start of clinical. Reinforce to your students that diversity is not a barrier to providing safe patient care, however interventions may require adjustments to demonstrate sensitivity to patient needs. Patience and respect of,differences in the patient-nurse relationship will result in trust, and better outcomes.

### CULTURAL, RACIAL AND ETHNIC DIVERSITY AMONG THE STAFF

Along with patients, nurses and other members of the health care team at the agency may also be diverse. Many physicians, nurses and caregivers have emigrated from other countries, and it is essential that students use collaborative and respectful communication skills as they work alongside these professionals. Non-native English-speaking individuals will be encountered, and it may be difficult for students to understand them. Students must ask for clarification if they are unsure about information that has been shared with them to ensure the safe delivery of care.

### DIVERSITY AMONG YOUR STUDENTS

Your clinical group may be comprised of students who are non-native English speakers, are racially or ethnically diverse, or identify as lesbian, gay, bisexual, transgender or queer (LGBTQ). Diversity in your clinical group is a very desirable situation and provides an opportunity for students to expand their knowledge and sensitivity to the needs of others via their peers. If a student was educated abroad they may not be fluent in the English language or could be difficult to understand creating a potential communication barrier. Verify that students understand directions that are given by asking them to verbalize their understanding of a plan of care for their patient. Personal beliefs and values embraced by students may present barriers to providing patient care. Students must realize that nurses are non-judgmental and provide care to all which can supersede their own belief systems.

### DIVERSITY AMONG PATIENTS

This may be the first time a student ever encountered diversity. This will increase anxiety, adding a further element of uncertainty to their knowledge base and skills. Encourage students to seek your assistance if questions arise. If challenges related to diversity occur during clinical, all students may learn from the encounter when discussed privately in post-conference. If you observe a situation where a student is hesitant to provide patient care due to their belief system, you must have a private discussion about their decision to become a nurse.

### DIVERSITY RELATED TO GENDER, AGE AND SEXUAL ORIENTATION

Male students are currently a minority in nursing programs and among licensed professional nurses (Buerhaus et al., 2017). If male student nurses are in a clinical group, be prepared to potentially encounter barriers during their clinical experience. You must advocate for their learning in a respectful manner to the staff or patient. If it is not possible, then consciously seek other opportunities for male students to gain a missed experience.

Muslim females may not permit a male student to care for them, which may be a learning barrier in labor and delivery. For modesty reasons or religious beliefs there may be objections to a male caregiver catheterizing a female patient. Inversely, but less often, some males patients will prefer a male caregiver to provide personal care. Seek alternatives to assure equity in the student's experience.

Generational barriers may also occur. When a student is assigned a patient their own age it may cause embarrassment for the patient or both during the provision of personal care. When a young student is assigned to an elderly patient, the patient may have concerns about trusting their care to a young student, believing they are too inexperienced.

Student nurses that encounter patients who identify as lesbian, gay, bisexual, transgender or queer (LGBTQ) must acknowledge that a patient identifies themselves with a specific group for their sexual identity. Be available to discuss any student concerns or feelings about caring for patients in this population prior to their encounter to educate and decrease anxiety if it exists. Students must demonstrate care for all patients without judgment or bias.

## RESPECT FOR CULTURAL OR RELIGIOUS PREFERENCES

Patients encountered in clinical may have preferences that are unfamiliar to your students, and even yourself. These experiences may include physical, spiritual, religious and nutritional practices.

### CONCERN ABOUT A LOVED ONE

Most health care agencies have implemented relaxed limitations on the number of visitors allowed in a room along with expanded visiting hours to be more welcoming to all. Family and significant others exhibit their concern and involvement in a variety of ways. We have observed individuals of Middle Eastern, Asian, and Hispanic ethnicities among groups who wish to continually remain with loved ones who are hospitalized. When certain treatments or personal care are being provided by the student, visitors may be asked to step out of the room. Be prepared to provide reassurance to the visitors, acknowledging any concerns that may accompany this request.

### PAIN MANAGEMENT

Non-traditional pain management techniques commonly practiced in other cultures may be unfamiliar, or concerning, to students. Examples such as cupping, coining and acupuncture that are used by Asian cultures for pain relief may be mistaken for physical abuse (Vitale & Prashad, 2017). The student nurse may note skin alterations during the documentation of an assessment. Other cultural groups perceive pain and its management differently, including their refusal for the administration of pain medications. If students verbalize their concerns to you, discussion about these observations will expand their knowledge of alternative non-pharmacologic pain management interventions.

### DIETARY RESTRICTIONS

Students must be aware of any dietary restrictions and food preferences of their patient. A family member may bring in a favorite dish, a customary food or "health food". If this conflicts with the physician's treatment plan, have the student alert you or the nurse. Most health care agencies can honor food preferences, such as a "kosher" diet, practiced in the Jewish faith, or a vegetarian preference. If patients wish to use herbal products brought in from home, teach students to consult with their nurse; it may require communicating with the physician and can interfere with medications.

### RESPECT FOR OTHER TREATMENT CHOICES

Religious practices that students may view as non-traditional from their personal experiences may include the refusal of blood products by Jehovah's Witness patients (Mendes, 2015), fasting despite nutritional deficiencies, and a patient visit from a medicine man or other "healer". These examples may be viewed as harmful by a student, so reinforcement of sensitivity to the patient's choices is a teaching opportunity.

Students will discover that other cultures may not place the same value on daily bathing and caring for themselves. This may be challenging for the student to accept since cleanliness and hygiene are strongly advocated to prevent the spread of infection. Encouraging the maintenance of a clean environment to a patient may require your involvement and negotiation on a student's behalf. Engage the assigned nurse in this discussion too. Teach the students that patients have the right of refusal unless risk exists.

### TERMINAL ILLNESS AND DEATH

Cultural and religious practices vary greatly especially in response to terminal illness, death and dying. For some ethnic groups, it is preferred that family members be informed of terminal illness before the patient is told. Nurses and students need to be respectful of the traditions and allow them to occur whenever possible. Most agencies have diversity specialists or a staff member that may assist if you encounter a challenging situation related to death and dying.

### SCENARIO 8-1 DIVERSITY ON THE NURSING UNIT

Your students are caring for patients on an oncology and hospice unit. The hospital chaplain, Reverend Rick, makes rounds throughout the agency daily. Today he approaches you regarding a patient on the unit. Without violating patient privacy, he explains that a Middle Eastern man is dying, and his death is imminent. Reverend Rick further explains that when this occurs, there will be loud wailing from his family members and to not be alarmed.

Reverend Rick states "this grief response is common to this culture, and we must respect the family's practice during this difficult time". He advised that the patient's door remain closed, however, the noise may still seem loud and may be upsetting to the students, staff and other patients. You will:

- Privately provide your clinical group with this information, so they will not be upset in the event the death occurs during your clinical day.
- Initiate a discussion with the students regarding adjustments to their provision of nursing care for patients with varying cultural practices.
- Possibly consider an assignment including researching rituals and practices by other cultural groups related to death and dying.

The chaplain's recognition of the student nurses' importance to the team through information sharing is also an example of collaboration to achieve the best patient outcome and visibly demonstrates respect for other cultures and religions. Other interdisciplinary staff at the agency where you are assigned may provide other valuable educational opportunities for your students.

### REFERENCES

Buerhaus, P.I., Skinner, L.E., Auerbach, D.I., & Staiger, D.O. (2017). State of the registered nurse workforce as a new era of health reform emerges. Nursing Economics 35(5):229–237.

Mendes, A. (2015). Culture and religion in nursing: providing culturally sensitive care. *British Journal of Nursing* 24(8):459.

Vitale, S.A. & Prashad, T. (2017). Cultural awareness: Coining and cupping. *International Archives of Nursing and Health Care* 3(3): 1-3. doi.org/10.23937/2469–5823/1510080.

The evaluation of students
# Nine

It is important to recognize that the evaluation of students' competency in the clinical setting must begin immediately, and measures for remediating deficient performance must be addressed quickly. Nursing programs conduct clinical experiences in semesters or quarters that can be any number of weeks, depending on the curriculum. Clinical hours may be six, eight or 12-hour shifts on one, or multiple days, per week. Therefore, determine early in the clinical rotation when a "midterm" evaluation meeting for every student should occur. Students really do want to know how they are progressing. Midterm evaluation is not just for the struggling student. Put your observations in a written format, which may or may not be provided to you by your nursing program.

## DOCUMENTATION

Students who are struggling to meet objectives during the clinical experience, need to be informed quickly both verbally and in writing. Lead faculty must also be notified at this time. This is the opportunity to arrange for a student to participate in remediation activities. You must not delay and wait, for, as mentioned, the semester quickly passes. Each nursing program has a process to document performance. Your written documentation must be clear and include any recommendations for the student who is at risk for failure, so they may have a fair opportunity to improve their performance.

## REMEDIATION

Remediation is utilized whenever a student is unable to demonstrate safe patient care, follow policy and procedures, or meet the course outcomes for the clinical rotation outlined in the syllabus. Examples include: A student who draws up medication incorrectly, performs injections in an unsafe manner, or is not prepared to discuss safe patient care. Your intervention is required in these instances. Communicating information to a student about their unsatisfactory progress is never easy. The goal is to constructively and respectfully communicate to the student a remediation plan based on your observations of their performance.

### *THE REMEDIATION PLAN*

Document instances you are concerned about including date, time, and a detailed factual description of the event to initiate the remediation process. You must provide time and opportunity for correction, with a definitive date for improvement. This requires a student to spend time in the skills laboratory for practice, or possibly submit a written assignment about a topic where the knowledge deficit exists. The student must sign the remediation form acknowledging they understand that not following these recommendations or unsuccessfully remediating the skill or knowledge deficit, will result in failure of the clinical course. This statement should be included in your communication to them. The accountability lies with the student to improve. Familiarize yourself with the school's communication process for sharing information to the lead faculty and the skills laboratory coordinator when a student requires remediation.

### SKILLS REMEDIATION PROCESS

Other instructors may be overseeing the student's remediation efforts, making it very important for you to communicate your expectations clearly in writing. A copy of your notes is extremely helpful to guide the remediation process. The skills laboratory coordinator will provide you with feedback, so you can subsequently observe if improvement has occurred. Remediation provides a student with the best chance for success and demonstrates that you implemented program policy. Your actions indicating that a student was advised of opportunities to improve performance, but remained unsuccessful, will uphold a student failure.

### CLINICAL FAILURE

It is imperative that you have time to observe improvement in a struggling student. You must provide the student with a fair and timely chance to prove that they are meeting the course objectives. Many students will improve their clinical skills when informed and given the opportunity. However, some students even with additional assistance and remediation may remain unsuccessful. In these instances, failure is the only option. Communicating regularly with the lead faculty when you have a student in jeopardy of failure is essential. They should offer support to both the student and you during this difficult situation, including their attendance at a meeting when the clinical failure is communicated. Providing the opportunity for open communication with the student that includes respectful dialogue, is mandatory in this uncomfortable and difficult situation.

## STUDENT APPEALS

Students are provided the option to appeal failures per college and nursing program policies. Review appeal policies approved by the nursing program. If you are asked to attend a formal grade appeal hearing, it will cause you anxiety and possibly make you feel inadequate as an instructor. However, your detailed and factual documentation of a student's performance will support your expert conclusion and can prevent an appeal from progressing to a hearing. Concise documentation includes: Dates, times, relevant statements and observations by yourself, or other staff members at the agency who observed deficient behaviors. Include specific details of meetings with the student, your discussion about their lack of progress, and the outcome of any remediation plan. Demonstrating that you provided a student with an adequate opportunity to improve their clinical performance, but that they still were not successful, will support your decision for a failure. Again, work with the program faculty lead to assist with your preparation.

## WEEKLY CLINICAL PROFICIENCY AND PROGRESSION (CPP) TOOL

If you are not provided with an evaluation tool by the nursing program, we have developed a framework to guide you week by week during the clinical experience. Form 9A, the Weekly Clinical Proficiency and Progression (CPP) Tool is a comprehensive, but not all-inclusive, list of behaviors that you can note during your student encounters. It may be adapted for your specific clinical experience to track your observations. Ideally you will use the other tracking documents provided in this book to compile information to add to the CPP Tool related to your students' performance.

The CPP Tool is intended to serve as a guide when you are reflecting about the activities and performance of each student during the clinical day. Make a copy for each student and keep daily and weekly anecdotal notes. For students who are not demonstrating the described behaviors, this is a trigger for you to begin more thorough documentation of your observations. Use a calendar to track clinical events sequentially. As an expert nurse, you will quickly observe if a student is struggling in the clinical setting, sometimes as early as the second or third encounter with them. Documentation of student performance must be handled as thoroughly as you would when providing care for a patient. This will assure you have a defensible response to challenges about a failure and ensure a fair assessment of student performance.

### SCENARIO 9-1 REMEDIATION OF STUDENT PERFORMANCE

Your student, Emily, will perform a dressing change on her patient. Last week she also performed a dressing change. It was her first time; she was so nervous and needed a lot of guidance and prompts along the way. Today you will look for improvements in her performance.

The dressing change order is for an abdominal wound to be irrigated with sterile normal saline and packed with wet gauze and covered with 4x4 pads and a large abdominal dressing and taped with silk tape.

You assess her preparedness and Emily says that she needs to bring more 4x4 pads. She can explain all steps correctly. Emily seems more confident than last week.

You stand close to the bed as Emily performs the dressing change. You observe, being ready to step in with guidance or correction. Emily has the following difficulties during the procedure:

- She tugs at the current dried dressing causing her patient pain
- When you suggest she wet the dressing with saline, Emily pours too much and wets the patients bed

You reassure the patient that Emily will put clean dry sheets on the bed. Emily removes the dressing and throws it away. When she redresses the wound, Emily makes several mistakes:

- She pours too much saline on the gauze dressings
- She contaminates the wound when packing it
- She drops a couple of 4x4s on the floor
- She forgets to date the dressing

After the procedure you review Emily's performance with her, telling her that she needs to seek remediation in the skills laboratory to practice her dressing changes. You write up a formal remediation plan that includes the date, time, and description of the event. Emily is given a copy which states clinical failure will occur if she does not successfully remediate to improve her clinical performance.

You thoroughly document the event in your anecdotal notes, adding to last week's notes on her first dressing change and noting that the remediation process was initiated. Notify the lead faculty member of Emily's poor performance and that you have sent her for remediation. You may utilize the CPP Tool, Form 9A in the Appendix, to guide you.

Emily successfully attends the skills laboratory remediation and has improved her dressing change skills. Two weeks later you assign Emily a patient with a wound dressing. This time she can successfully change the dressing without making any errors.

You are the clinical instructor for a group of students in their first medical-surgical rotation. Kayleigh is a student who has been sent to the skills laboratory on two occasions for errors related to several poor techniques that may have resulted in patient harm described below:

- During week two Kayleigh was unable to maintain sterility while donning gloves to insert a urinary catheter; she states, "well everything is still clean, right?"

- After two failed attempts to correct her technique, you privately discuss the error with the student and document in detail that she is required to spend time in the skills laboratory for remediation of the procedure prior to the next clinical day. Urinary catheter insertion had been taught during the previous semester. Kayleigh is visibly upset and states "I don't have time to make an extra trip to campus!" You remind her that this is a requirement for her to complete in order to return to clinical.

- During week three an opportunity for Kayleigh to don sterile gloves again occurred while performing a central line dressing change which you observe.

- The student again does not don the gloves properly during this encounter and contaminates the sterile field; you obtain a new dressing kit and complete the procedure yourself, and ensure patient comfort, waiting to discuss the error with Kayleigh after exiting the room.

- You document a second remediation plan for Kayleigh, describing in detail so the skills laboratory instructors could again work with her to help her improve her technique; in your notes you indicate that further instances of the student's inability to maintain sterile technique will result in a clinical failure; as you present this to her privately she begins to cry and states, "you are not being fair to me!" Add the student's behavior and statement to your notes.

- You calmly explain to the student that she must meet the objectives for the clinical experience as outlined in the course syllabus, one of them stating that she can provide safe care.
- After the second incident you contact the lead faculty to inform them of the student's status in the clinical rotation: She is not meeting the objectives currently and may be at risk for a clinical failure.
- Provide the lead faculty with a copy of your documentation. The student may seek out this individual while she is on campus, especially since she is upset.
- During the fifth week of the clinical rotation, following Kayleigh's second remediation in the laboratory she again cannot maintain sterility of the urinary catheter kit. You stop the procedure, ensure the patient's comfort, and ask the nurse to insert the catheter.
- You advise Kayleigh that you will be having her research sterile technique on the internet and not participate in further direct care of patients for the remainder of the day. She begins to cry.
- Immediately contact the lead faculty via phone or email to advise them you are recommending a clinical failure for Kayleigh. Document the incident thoroughly along with the behavior and statements made by the student.
- Arrange for a meeting on campus with the lead faculty or another member in attendance when you inform the student they have not met the clinical outcomes of the course and have failed.

Overall ensure that your documentation throughout remains factual, include the student's statements, and summarize events as accurately as possible with a defined timeline that contains evidence of attempts for the student to succeed. Always use your lead faculty as a guide when you encounter a challenging student situation—they are there to assist.

Accountability, collaboration, and professional
relationships

# Ten

As a nursing instructor you are accountable to provide the best learning experience possible for you students. Nursing staff must understand that you and the students are guests in the agency and must not be included in staffing assignments. Communicate that you are willing to help; however, there may be limitations. You must follow agency policies and procedures that pertain to nursing students. Your nursing program will specify guidelines that outline what students may do during clinical.

One example of a limitation may be if a nurse asks a student to insert a urinary catheter and the student has not been taught or performed the skill in laboratory. You must communicate that they cannot do this. When you or the student are asked to perform a task that you are not comfortable with, or nursing policy does not permit, refuse and communicate the rationale. Another example is when a nurse wants a student to follow a pain medication schedule that they state is allowed per the physician, but the medication orders do not align with that schedule. You must teach the students to always follow physician orders. If staff are performing a wound care procedure and the orders are not clear, you must refuse to complete it, or ask for written clarification. Do not let the student perform a procedure until clarity is obtained. When you encounter a situation you are unfamiliar with you may also seek assistance from other agency resources for a later opportunity.

### INTERDISCIPLINARY COLLABORATION

Most acute care agencies have nurse educators or a clinical nurse specialist that you may contact to help you and your students provide safe and appropriate care. In smaller agencies a manager may serve in a dual role as supervisor and educator and are valuable resources too.

As earlier discussed, other specialty nurses you may wish to develop relationships with may include wound care and ostomy nurses. They are very knowledgeable and welcome the opportunity to educate students. Other examples may be advanced practice nurses that serve in the role of a primary care provider and can demonstrate more complex assessment skills to your students as they visit patients. Their presence will vary based on the type of agency you are assigned too.

Pharmacist and case managers are also great resources. They may be available to speak to your students in post-conference about their role in patient care and education. These interactions familiarize a student with the broad continuum of care and promotes collegiality among the interdisciplinary team.

### UNIT COLLABORATION

The nursing unit manager is an excellent resource to you. There may also be a charge nurse assigned that can be more accessible to you in the event a procedural issue or incident arises on the unit and you are not sure how to proceed. An example is if the narcotic count is not accurate when you and your student attempt to remove a dose for a patient. A responsible staff member or manager will guide you to the correct process of documenting the shortage, permitting you to move on with other patient care activities. It is also a learning opportunity for the student.

## NURSING PROGRAM COLLABORATION

Student performance issues including violations related to program policies may be initially handled by you if they are minor and are quickly corrected by the student. If they are repeated or rise to a more serious level as discussed in Chapter Nine, it is highly advisable to contact the lead faculty member or your program administrator for guidance as soon as possible. A minor example is when a student continually violates the published dress code. Ask the lead faculty member if you are allowed to send the student home after a second infraction occurs. A major example is when a student has an incident of unsafe care. You may stop a student in the middle of a procedure if they are demonstrating unsatisfactory performance and make a referral for remediation.

After you have gained more experience in your role as a clinical instructor you will feel more confident in your decisions. Always know that the lead faculty member and administrators are accountable to you, and the success of students. You should feel supported when you bring forth a concern.

## RELATIONSHIP BARRIERS ON THE NURSING UNIT

Incivility, lateral violence or bullying in nursing practice are behaviors, although unpleasant, that require discussion. A great deal of information is available about these topics in the nursing literature for your review. Observations such as eye-rolling, ignoring requests for information, or other efforts to sabotage student success are examples of inappropriate behavior. A specific example is when a staff member belittles your student in front of a patient or family member, accusing them of not performing care, when in fact, they did. Hopefully you will never encounter incivility, lateral violence, or bullying of your students during the clinical experience.

You may encounter staff members who are difficult to collaborate with, and there may be instances when you cannot prevent assigning your student to work with them. Do not avoid assigning a patient with a chest tube or other interesting health issues to a student because of the nurse caring for the patient. In these instances, be extra diligent while communicating the student's responsibility for provision of care to the nurse. Be readily available if the nurse has any questions or concerns during the clinical day.

You need to be proactive to prevent these instances from occurring or escalating. When they occur, the behavior must be identified, and the nurse manager alerted to avoid further instances. Ideally, a frank discussion between the involved staff member and you related to respectful communication with students is warranted. Once on their own, students will undoubtedly encounter colleagues who have different work practices and attitudes, but patient care still must be accomplished.

### PROMOTING POSITIVE RELATIONSHIPS

When you demonstrate to the nurses on your unit your willingness to help them by actively completing patient care with your students and assisting whenever feasible, this builds rapport and trust, and the staff are eager to help you as well. Many nurses enjoy teaching and are willing to share information and knowledge. Observant nurses will notice when you are getting behind with tasks and may offer to pass the medications with the student or observe a dressing change for you. In those instances, you can use your judgment and allow it knowing that the nurse will report back to you about student performance.

Expect that the nurses are watching your students when you are not around and will report concerns to you. Elicit input from nursing staff working with students to verify any problems they may have observed. This information may assist you as you prepare to evaluate your student. When your clinical rotation ends, a thank you gesture may be appropriate, for working with student nurses can be stressful for staff. A thank you card, and if possible, some bagels or cookies are usually welcome. This gesture can solidify future professional relationships between you and the staff.

### SCENARIO 10-1 ACCOUNTABILITY AND PROFESSIONAL RELATIONSHIPS

Your student, Nicole, approaches you and asks if she can administer her patient's pain medication. You check the MAR and notice that it is not time to give the medication. The order reads Hydromorphone 2 mg every four hours IVP for severe pain. The student states that the nurse told her she could give the dose an hour early. You accompany Nicole to talk to the nurse. The nurse states that the doctor is "aware that the patient is getting her doses an hour early sometimes". You will privately:

• State to the nurse that you will be happy to have Nicole administer the medication when it is due.
• Remind the nurse that students must follow the physician orders as written and respectfully inform her that you wish for the student to abide by the time interval as a learning opportunity.

- Respectfully ask the nurse if she believes the physician's order should be modified if the patient is routinely requesting their pain medication early.
- Inform the nurse that they may wish to administer the medication themselves and to inform the student if the physician's order changes.

Afterwards, discuss the incident with Nicole:

- "Do you understand why you are unable to administer the medication early?"
- "Why do you think the patient may be wanting the pain medication sooner?"
- "Do you think this is something that should discussed with the physician?"
- Explain that nurses have responsibility and accountability to follow physician orders as written.
- Stress that nurses should always advocate for the patient and notify the physician when patients' concerns or condition warrant changes in the plan of care.

After the students leave the unit for the day, assess if this encounter has created a strained professional relationship. Reiterate the student's role while in clinical with the nurse, and your expectation that they always follow policy, procedures and physician orders as written to reinforce student awareness of patient safety.

# Appendix 4C

**SO YOU** WANT TO TEACH **CLINICAL?**
A Guide for New Nursing Clinical Instructors

**EXAMPLE 4C**

## TYPICAL CLINICAL DAY
*(Times are approximate)*

| Time Frame | Expected Clinical Activity |
| --- | --- |
| 0700 | Arrive on unit ready for patient assignments. Gain access to med room to write down medications you will be giving. |
| 0730 | Get report from your RN, and her phone number. Greet your patient. Look up Medications. Give Insulin + 0800 Meds |
| 0800 | Give AM care. Begin Assessment. Check all IV sites and tubes and catheters. Plan your care – May begin to document. |
| 0815 | Be ready to pass 0900 medications. Follow the 5 rights of medication administration. |
| 0900–1100 | Chart VS and physical assessments in EMR. Prepare to perform any treatments with Instructor. Read the EMR. Check morning labs. Review EMR for new orders, and gather data. Teach your patient. |
| 1100–1145 | Lunch – students will report off to their RN or whoever is covering for them. |
| 1145–1250 | Reassess patient upon return from lunch (note changes in EMR). Have charting (progress note) ready for instructor review. Write progress note on chart. |
| 1215 | Prepare for 1300 meds. Finish all documentation in EMR and any patient care tasks. |
| 1300 | Give 1300 meds. Prepare to leave the unit. Check that your patient is comfortable and safe with call light within reach. |
| 1340 | Report off to your RN and let the patient care assistant know you are leaving the unit. |
| 1345–1445 | Post–conference |

Appendix 4D

**SO YOU** WANT TO TEACH **CLINICAL?**
A Guide for New Nursing Clinical Instructors

**Patient Care Type**

| STUDENTS | RESPIRATORY DIAGNOSIS | ABDOMINAL SURGERY | GYN SURGERY | PATIENT WITH OSTOMY | HEAD AND NECK SURGERY | DVT | OTHER |
|---|---|---|---|---|---|---|---|
| #1 | COPD | Colon resection | Abd hysterectomy | | | Left leg | |
| #1 | | Whipple | Bladder suspension | | Trach | | Post op wound infection |
| #3 | COPD | Appendectomy | | Ileostomy | Thyroidectomy | | |
| #4 | Asthma | Ostomy reversal | | | Trach | Right Leg | |

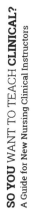

# SO YOU WANT TO TEACH CLINICAL?
A Guide for New Nursing Clinical Instructors

## Clinical, Activity & Assignment Calendar
*Fill out with medication administration and any of the assignments or activities.*

| STUDENT | **Clinical Dates:** | | | | | | | | |
| --- | --- | --- | --- | --- | --- | --- | --- | --- | --- |
| | Sept. 14 | Sept. 21 | Sept. 28 | Oct. 4 | Oct. 11 | Oct. 18 | Oct. 25 | Nov. 1 |
| 1 | Meds | OR Rotation | Meds | 2 Patients | Meds | 2 Patients | Meds | 2 Patients |
| 2 | Meds | 2 Patients | Meds | OR Rotations | Meds | 2 Patients | Meds | 2 Patients |
| 3 | 2 Patients | Meds | 2 Patients | Meds | OR Rotation | Meds | 2 Patients | Meds |
| 4 | OR Rotation | Meds | 2 Patients | Meds | 2 Patients | Meds | 2 Patients | Meds |
| 5 | Meds | 2 Patients | Meds | 2 Patients | Meds | OR Rotation | Meds | 2 Patients |
| 6 | 2 Patients | Meds | OR Rotation | Meds | 2 Patients | Meds | 2 Patients | Meds |

Appendix 4G

# SO YOU WANT TO TEACH CLINICAL?
A Guide for New Nursing Clinical Instructors

## EXAMPLE 4G

## Patient Information Chart

This form is where you put information you as the instructor gathered from the EMR and the nursing staff. It is a good idea to use different colored ink for pertinent info like code status, isolation or treatments. Add another color for any information the student adds as the day progresses i.e. their assessment of lung and bowel sounds. This document will help you when grading care plans. You can refer to it to ensure the proper nursing diagnoses were used based on the data you have listed. It also helps you jog your memory of the patient when reading papers since no patient names are used only patient demographics.

| STUDENTS | PATIENT | PATIENT |
|---|---|---|
| #1<br>JP | Rm 302 76y/o(F) Dx: TIA Hx: T2DM, HTN, Breast CA R Mastectomy, BS q 6h w/cov, A+Ox2. Confusion VS 170/94, 68, 20 O, Sat 95% RA Lytes, CBC today PBS 206 BRP Fall Risk | |
| #2<br>KR | Rm 324 54y/o(M) Dx: Leukemia Receiving Chemotherapy. Strict Handwashing. Bleeding Precautions Daily CBC w/Diff to receive Blood and Platelets Hgb 7.9 Platelets 10 VS 120/80 100 24 37P Pt receiving NS + Baking soda mouth rinses qid Bone marrow bx drsg | |
| #3 | | |

Appendix 4H

**SO YOU** WANT TO TEACH **CLINICAL?**
A Guide for New Nursing Clinical Instructors

**EXAMPLE 4H**

## Student Clinical Day Progress Report

| STUDENTS | ROOM # | VS | I&O | TXS | PAIN ASMT | POC | PHYS ASMT | OTHER ASMT | OTHER ASMT | ORAL MEDS | INJECT | IV | IVPB | NOTES |
|---|---|---|---|---|---|---|---|---|---|---|---|---|---|---|
| #1 JP | 302 | 1710/P94 68 20 | ✓ | | 0800 0/10 1500 0/10 | ✓ ④ | 1100 ④ | Neuro ③ | | ④ | Insulin ③ | hung ③ | | Needs practice drawing up insulin |
| #2 KR | 324 | 120/80 100 24 37° | 1 Unit Blood Platelets | ✓ Bone Marrow Drsg | 0900 0/10 1300 2/10 | ✓ ② | 1300 ④ | | | ④ | | | hung ④ | Needed extra help with POC |
| #3 | 315 | | | | | | | | | | | | | OR Rotation |
| #3 | 314 | | | | | | | | | | | | | |
| #4 | 301 | | | | | | | | | | | | | |
| #4 | 307 | | | | | | | | | | | | | |

POC = Plan of care  TXs=Treatments  Asmt=Assessments
Grading: 5= proficient; 4= good; 3= fair; 2= needs improvement; 1= unacceptable (may need remediation)

Appendix 4I

## SO YOU WANT TO TEACH **CLINICAL?**
A Guide for New Nursing Clinical Instructors

### Skills Checklist
(You can add or change any of these boxes to match the skills available on your unit.)

| STUDENTS | OI | STRAIGHT CATH | CATHETER INSERT | REMOVE CATHETER | BLADDER SCAN | CBI | IRRIGATE CATHETER | ISOLATION | ORAL SUCTION | TRACH CARE | TRACH SUCTION | DRESSING CHANGE | OSTOMY CARE | CHEST TUBE |
|---|---|---|---|---|---|---|---|---|---|---|---|---|---|---|
| 1 | | | | | | | | | | | | | | |
| 2 | | | | | | | | | | | | | | |
| 3 | | | | | | | | | | | | | | |
| 4 | | | | | | | | | | | | | | |
| 5 | | | | | | | | | | | | | | |
| 6 | | | | | | | | | | | | | | |
| 7 | | | | | | | | | | | | | | |

## Concept Map

JP
**Name**

---

### Nursing Diagnosis # 1 Risk for Fall/Injury

**Supporting Data:**

Recent TIA
Occasional confusion
Lisinopri
Head CT, B/P 174/94 P68, R 20 PaO2 95%
Fall risk

**Short Term Goal:**

Pt will not experience any falls during the shift

**Nursing Interventions:**

RN will
1. Instruct patient to call for assistance when getting up.
2. Monitor for confusion, and re-orientate.
3. Initiate bed alarm.
4. Place personal items within reach of patient.

**Evaluation:** Met/Not Met

**Revision:**

None

---

### Diagnosis: TIA

**PMH:**

Type 2 Diabetes, Hypertension, Breast Cancer

**PSH:**

Right radical mastectomy

---

### Nursing Diagnosis # 3 Ineffective health maintenance

**Supporting Data:**

B/P 174/94 P68, BS 206
Widowed lives alone, limited support system

**Short Term Goal:**

Arrangements for post-discharge care and support
1. Assess patient's level of knowledge related to their care needs.
2. If feasible, discussion with family or friend regarding medication education and administration.
3. Partner with discharge planning or care management to arrange for home care visits or alternative living situation.

---

### Nursing Diagnosis # 2 Altered Tissue Perfusion

**Supporting Data:**

Alert and oriented x 2–3, occasional confusion about being in the hospital
Elevated (B/P 174/94), P 68, R 20, PaO2—95% on room air
Lisinopri

**Short Term Goal:**

Improved Cognition, decreased B/P during the shift

**Nursing Interventions:**

1. Neuro checks every 4 hours
2. VS monitoring every 4 hours, compare to baseline VS data
3. BS with sliding scale insulin every 6 hours if indicated
4. Safety checks every 2 hours
5. Administer anti-hypertensives as ordered, hold if vital sign parameters fall below recommended range: <110/60 or pulse 60 bpm, or as physician recommends.

**Evaluation:** Met/Not Met

**Revision:**

Notify the MD of continued elevated blood pressure

Appendix 6A

 **SO YOU** WANT TO TEACH **CLINICAL?**
A Guide for New Nursing Clinical Instructors

**EXAMPLE 6A**

## Medication Administration Tracking Record
*(Fill in times to reflect your clinical day)*

| STUDENT | MEDICATIONS DUE AT: | | | |
|---------|------|------|--------|------|
| | 0800 | 1000 | 11–1200 | 1300 |
| **1**<br><br>JP | Metformin PO<br>Aspart Insulin Coverage SC | Lisinopril PO<br>Tamoxifin PO | Aspart Insulin Coverage SC | |
| **2**<br><br>KR | Reglan IVPB<br>Mycostatin<br>Swish + Swallow | Allopurinol PO<br>Valtrex PO<br>Bactrim PO | | |
| **3** | | | | |
| **4** | | | | |

Appendix 6B

**SO YOU** WANT TO TEACH **CLINICAL?**
A Guide for New Nursing Clinical Instructors

## Student Medication Preparation

JP     Mrs. M     Oct. 8
**Name**     **Patient Initials**     **Date**

| DRUG AND CLASSIFICATION | DRUG ACTION | REASON FOR ADMINISTERING | DOSE ROUTE | RELEVANT LABS | PATIENT LABS | NURSING IMPLICATIONS |
|---|---|---|---|---|---|---|
| Aspart Insulin Exogenous Insulin Antidiabetic | Facilitates passage of glucose across cell membranes. Promotes conversion of glucose to glycogen in the liver | Type 2 DM | 5 units SC | Glucose | FBS 206 | Administer 5-10 minutes before meals Monitor for hypoglycemia |
| Lisinopril Ace Inhibitor Antihypertensive | Suppresses angiotension-renin-aldosterone system | Hypertension | 10mg PO | Renal function | Not ordered | Take BP prior to giving Monitor BP Assess for edema |
| | | | | | | |
| | | | | | | |
| | | | | | | |

# Appendix 7A

**SO YOU** WANT TO TEACH **CLINICAL?**
A Guide for New Nursing Clinical Instructors

---

### Alternative Experience: Visit to OR
*The student will answer the following questions and submit in a short paper after their OR visit experience.*

..........................................................................................................................................

**①** Describe the process during pre—op holding for obtaining informed consent

**②** Describe the following roles of the following personnel:
  A. Surgeon
  B. Scrub Nurse
  C. Surgical Tech
  D. Circulating Nurse
  E. Anesthesiologist/CRNA

**③** Provide your understanding of sterile field

**④** Describe the nurse's role in the PACU

**⑤** List the criteria for discharge from PACU

**⑥** Provide a nursing diagnosis for each area of the operative experience

---

Page numbers in **bold** refer to boxes

Printed in the United States
by Baker & Taylor Publisher Services